Rodolphe
In collaborati
Betty Dandrieux and

The
Healing Power of
Essential Oils

Fragrance Secrets for Everyday Use
This handbook is a compact reference work
on the effects and applications of 248 essential oils
for health, fitness, and well-being

LOTUS LIGHT
SHANGRI-LA

1st English edition 1996
© by Lotus Light Publications
Box 325, Twin Lakes, WI 53181
The Shangri-La Series is published in cooperation
with Schneelöwe Verlagsberatung, Federal Republic of Germany
© 1990 reserved by Windpferd Verlagsgesellschaft mbH, Aitrang
All rights reserved
Title of the original edition *Les huiles essentielles*
Translation by Samsara Amato Duex
English translation edited by Christine M. Grimm
Cover design by Wolfgang Jünemann—based on an illustration by Berthold Rodd
Photos: © by *Photocentre de production Sanoflore (France)*
ISBN 0-941524-89-2

Printed in the USA

TABLE OF CONTENTS

It has long been known that the subtle element of plants—the aroma of the flowers—is contained and concentrated within essential oils. These oils, which actually contain "the power of light," embody the principles of the transitory acknowledged to be just as necessary as the indispensable principles of life. Here we come up against the vital forces of alchemy in the creation process.

These aromatic plant essences offer an infinite variety of possibilities for regeneration, revitalizing and healing. They open up an extraordinary field of activity for both prevention and therapy in human beings.

Foreword

This book introduces us to knowledge of the healing power of plants, particularly their active extracts, the essential oils. Here you will also find the effects of well-known essences like cypress, lavender, patchouli, sandalwood, ylang-ylang ...

This method can be understood by every reader willing to deal with the relationship between symptom and illness on the one hand and medicine on the other hand. The healing power of essential oils is ultimately dependent on a person's willingness to acknowledge them as medication. This leads us to self-treatment without eliminating the need for the advice of a specialist, who can diagnose the illness or the nature of the terrain. Once this has been clarified, an independent path can be followed. Using the table of contents and the index, afflicted persons can determine their own aromatherapy and prepare their own mixtures and solutions. Every illness is the sign of an inner or outer imbalance, of which the afflicted person must become conscious. If the essential oil is to be effective, the person must inevitably also examine his or her lifestyle and way of life, including eating habits, making sure that these are harmonious.

Dr. Alain Ringger

Introduction

From morning until night, smells are part of our daily lives. Some are pleasing and invigorating, others nauseating or poisonous. Yet, a social taboo discriminates against the sense of smell. Sight and hearing are rated the highest; then comes the sense of taste, so very important to our modern gourmets; with its relationship to the body and its less socialized sensations, the sense of touch is more problematic. At the bottom of the list is the sense of smell, which only imparts certain generally good or bad sensations. Its lower status is already expressed in the fact that we have a difficult time making precise statements about smells. We lack the words to precisely describe a smell: all of which expresses a feeling of impropriety that arises in various degrees of intensity.

Old German had some forty words designating different types of smell. The dearth of expressions prevalent today in English in this domain suggests that this sense has degenerated. Even scientific research is affected by this taboo: smell is by far the least investigated of our senses. Only in the past few years has fundamental research groundwork taken place. As a result, we have increasingly discovered the wealth of impressions which this sense can inform us about and how strongly it connects us with the rest of the world.

We are also beginning to understand that smell is one of the keys to an awareness of the ecological equilibrium between the plant kingdom, animal kingdom and human beings. Through the sense of smell, a multitude of information is exchanged, for which human beings have become less and less receptive following the atrophy of their olfactory sense.

When a plant reaches the climax of its development, it flowers and releases fragrance into the air. This means it communicates with the animal world and attracts, for example, insects which make pollination, fructification and therefore the survival of its species possible. Because the plant's pollen is a food, the insects also benefit from the transaction. Since bees turn pollen into honey, human beings also benefit. In the animal kingdom, smells are the major source of information. They are essential to the survival of the species, providing information about food, enemies and possible dangers. During the fertility period, they stimulate the reproductive hormones and mating. This latter function is apparently suppressed in human beings, although the popularity of perfumes, most of which are artificially manufactured, is an indication of efforts in this direction.

The subtle language of smell should be rediscovered. In the past, the value of smells was related to both health and spirituality; this is where the expression "odor of sanctity" has its origins. In ancient times, pleasant fragrances were the food of the gods.

When we are in good health, we smell good; our bodily fluids and perspiration have an agreeable odor. Conversely, when we are ill, we develop a bad smell. One example of this is perspiration caused by gardening, which smells pleasant; but perspiration caused by stress has a disagreeable odor. The relationship to our emotional state is obvious, which is also verified by the Latin word "humor" for the body fluids. It is well known that saints give off an agreeable smell, and even at their moment of death, this pleasant fragrance can linger. These are just a few indications of what agreeable effects the aromas of plants may have in store for us.

Even though it is the least appreciated of our senses, the sense of smell is paradoxically the most refined. It has a very high perceptive ability. We can, for example, recognize and identify musk (a substance which is related to sexuality) up to a concentration of 0.000000000003 grams per cubic meter of air. The human being could be capable of differentiating up to ten thousand different smells and remembering them. The olfactory nerve ends directly in the higher centers of the brain, whereas information from the other four senses must first be processed in the thalamus before being directed towards the various zones of the brain. It is the rhinencephalic part of the brain which identifies and deciphers olfactory stimuli. Although we do not yet know how this occurs, one of its main functions appears to be to connecting the instinctual drives securing survival, originating in the paleocephalic brain, with the symbolic and conceptual functions of the neocephalic brain.

Through the course of the ages, the brain in the animal kingdom has continued to evolve, particularly in the mammals, to become most highly developed in the primates and in human beings. The paleocephalic brain (primitive brain) with the hypothalamus governs instinctual behavior pertaining to the survival and reproduction of the species. In a later stage of development, the mesocephalic brain (mid-brain) with the limbic system was formed. It is generally considered to be the center of affective behavior and plays an essential role in the development of long-term memory. It conveys the association of pleasant and unpleasant experiences in time and space and makes possible the development of emotions. Specifically in human beings, the neocephalic brain (cerebral cortex or neocortex) was the last section to evolve: this is where thought, language and consciousness have their origin.

Smells and the sense of smell therefore also act as the connection between the primitive brain with its animalistic survival instincts, the limbic system with its relationship to memory and emotions, and the neocortex, the seat of conscious thought and therefore those elements which are specifically human with our cultural and spiritual dimensions.

"The fundamental regulation mechanisms of the organism are characterized by complex cycles and interactions which extend far beyond the limits of the individual organism into the center of the surrounding environment".

(Joel de Rosnay)

Stress, fears, frustration, joy, pleasure and well-being all constantly influence the nervous, hormonal and energetic regulatory processes of our bodies. They therefore cause specific smells reflecting our physical, psychological, and overall state of health. Research has confirmed what the majority of peoples perceived throughout the various ages: smells reveal the essence of things, the souls of plants, animals and human beings. This also allows us to understand how smells from our environment can influence our regulative systems, our energy potential, and therefore our entire state of being.

It is up to each individual to rediscover and use the sense of smell, the sense which most directly connects us with the nature within us and around us.

As St. Hildegard of Bingen said:

"With the eyes, the human being perceives his path; with the nose, he understands it".

11

How to Use This Book

Because it is useful, I recommend that you read all of this book. But in order to profit from the application of essential oils, you should carefully study certain chapters in any case.

Chapters I and II introduce the reader to the relationship between human beings and the plant kingdom, as well as providing specific advice on preventive hygiene.

Chapters III, VI and VII are dedicated to the properties and characteristics of essential oils.

Chapters V and VI must be read before you attempt to make practical use of essential oils.

Paragraph 5 in chapter V explains how to use the therapeutic index in chapter VIII.

Please read:

a. Chapter VI (Internal Uses, 4. Preparation and Doses for Oral Use) when you want to prepare essential oils for internal use. Chapter V (How to Choose Essential Oils ...) gives you advice for making a preparation personally tailored to your own needs. The chart in Chapter VII (Table of Essential Oils ...) informs you about the common, rare and expensive essential oils. Chapter VIII (Therapeutic Index) indicates which essential oils are appropriate for specific symptoms or types of illness.

b. Chapter VI (The Many Types of External Uses) is arranged in categories and offers information on the external use of essential oils for inhalation or creation of perfumes or shampoos. A chart of common and rare essential oils can be found in Chapter VII.

c. Chapter VI (How to Flavor Baked Goods and Other Foods) and Chapter VII (Chart of Essential Oils) inform you on how to use essential oils in the kitchen.

Chapter I

Human Beings and the Plant Kingdom

The Use of Plants Goes Back to the Origin of Humanity

From the beginning of time, human beings have lived in a symbiotic relationship with plants. Plants provided food, clothing, shelter, fire, smoke, scents for funeral and sacred rites and remedies for healing. In addition to breeding of animals and farming, ancient civilizations on all the continents developed healing arts based on plants. One of the first western discourses on herbal medicine was written on papyrus scrolls in Egypt from the period 3000 years before Christ.

This natural form of therapy evolved throughout the ages. People knew in an intuitive, comprehensive and experiential way that relationships existed between plants, soil, human beings, the world and the cosmos. They were aware of the plants' medicinal properties and energetic values. This knowledge has largely been lost in modern times. Until just about 150 years ago, herbal medicine was the prevalent official medicine and most great physicians of the past were phytotherapists.

Modern Phytoaromatherapy

Herbal medicine and the use of plant essences for healing, currently undergoing a revival, are not merely a new fad. Instead, this is an expression of a growing disillusionment with chemical drugs and their many side-effects, compounded by their incomprehensible names and compositions on the one hand; and on the other, it points to the rediscovery of the multiple connections and laws of harmony which unite human beings with nature and the cosmos.

The Relationship Between Human Beings and Nature

Vegetable and animal species may be regarded as early evolutionary stages in the development of man: our distant ancestors as it were. They obey nature's biological and cosmic laws just like we do, but even better than we do.

This harmony between the plant kingdom and the human world is manifested in the fact that both are dependent on and complement each other. We see it at work, for example, in the most important of all vital functions: breathing. Human beings and animals inhale oxygen and breathe out carbon dioxide; plants take in carbon dioxide and give off oxygen. This well-known fact has far-reaching consequences for human life.

Today we know that plants contribute to the ionization of the air, mainly through the essential oils they release. In this context, the ionization of the air means the formation of the negatively charged oxygen molecules necessary for human life. The more ionized (negative ions) the air contains, the healthier and more vitalizing it is; the less ionized (positive ions), the greater the risk of susceptibility and poor health.

Various research studies have found evidence establishing that the aromatic compounds in plants have a constitution similar to that of the fluids in the tissue of the human body. This could explain the vivifying and harmonizing effect of aroma substances in plants. The relationship of our sense of smell with plants may be summed up as follows: smells we like benefit our health.

This harmony between plants and human beings is also expressed in other fields. Plants emit rays which have a positive effect on people. Each of us can verify this experience: we just have to think of the feeling of harmony and peace that we sense while walking in a forest, for example. The reverse is equally true. Our positive or negative attitudes towards plants can affect them in a positive or negative sense. No true gardener can deny that a plant looked after with care and love will grow to be stronger and more beautiful than the others. This also partly explains the mystery of "green thumb," or why some people's plants thrive so well compared to those of other people.

Try it for yourself: plant two seeds of the same plant in the earth. Water them alike, but pay more attention to one of them than the other by concentrating on it and talking to it. You will be astonished at the result.

This interaction also explains why many amateur gardeners find gardening a relaxing, harmonizing and rejuvenating activity.

The Anthroposophical Approach

The studies of Rudolph Steiner (1861-1925) have brought to light other interesting complementary aspects of the relationship between plants and human beings. One of these aspects is the three-part structure: human beings are made of three systems and these systems have their counterparts in plants.

1. The rhythmic system: Consisting of the respiratory and the circulatory system in human beings, it corresponds to the foliage of plants since this is where breathing and photosynthesis occur. The leaves and the essential oils extracted from them are particularly suited for respiratory, circulatory and heart complaints. A further analogy should be mentioned here: chlorophyll acts as a catalyst for photosynthesis and colors the leaves green. The color green is the color complementary to red. Green is the fluorescent color for the red in our blood, and red is the florescent color for green. It has been discovered that chlorophyll acts as a potent blood-regenerating substance (especially because it activates the production of red blood corpuscles) and a heart stimulant.

2. The neuro-sensory system: The human head corresponds to the roots of the plants. Many root extracts have a considerable effect on the brain and nervous system.

3. The metabolism: The functions of digestion, assimilation, excretion and reproduction in human beings correspond to the flowers and fruit of the plants. Seeds and blossoms generally have a beneficial effect on our digestion and metabolism.

The following diagram illustrates the interactions between human beings and plants:

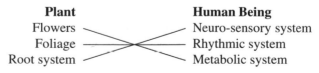

Plant	**Human Being**
Flowers	Neuro-sensory system
Foliage	Rhythmic system
Root system	Metabolic system

The diagram of the three-part structure of plants and human beings offers interesting perspectives from various vantage points. Although we will limit ourselves here to just one aspect, it provides an abundance of information and further suggestions for research.

The middle system (which is the foliage in plants and the rhythmic system in humans) is one of equilibrium and connection. It creates the relationship between the other two systems and can subdue or stimulate them as required. It connects what is above with what is below, terrestrial influences with cosmic influences, and gaseous states with solid and liquid states.

It is indeed our blood circulation and breathing that distribute life in our bodies, making exchanges possible, bringing energy and removing waste products. Breathing in particular is an excellent regulative system and an important element in the state of our health. We can consciously experience and influence it. Through breathing we can also come into contact with the invigorating aromas of the essential oils. These observations can also be extended in both of the following directions:

1. If we compare the earth with a large body, the zone with the Mediterranean climate is found in the middle part. This zone is most suited for the growth of the labiate plant family, which represent a large portion of the aromatic and medicinal plants. Nearly all labiates have a beneficial influence on the human rhythmic system. This analogy is not a coincidence: the Mediterranean areas are regions of equilibrium where the influence of the cosmos and the earth (climate, sunlight, soil) are equally distant from the poles and the equator.

In the Mediterranean zone, the cosmic forces of heat exert an extraordinary influence on the development of plants. A harmonious balance between their roots, leaves and flowers is created. In its position between the dry/hot or humid/hot climate of the equatorial zones and the dry/cold of the polar regions, the Mediterranean area enjoys a long summer and a short, rainy and cool winter. The summer heat and the special light found in Provence becomes embodied in the aromatic essences of its plant world. The inimitable fragrances of lavender and rosemary and the intoxicating aromas of the evergreen shrubs are created here. Essential oils are very rich in hydrogen, and, according to W. Pelikan, the essence of rosemary is the most hydrogenated substance known to man, for example. In turn, hydrogen is the substance most closely related to heat on the earth.

2. The effect of essential oils from the labiates on the human body is almost always on the respiratory and circulatory systems. This applies particularly to the areas around the respiratory organs, the lungs, the

solar plexus, the heart and the epigastrium. These parts of our bodies are centers of some of our psychological functions such as the self or the will which is usually placed at the level of the solar plexus, joy is located in the heart, anxiety can be found in the neck and epigastrium, etc. We also know that many labiates have an influence on the psyche. Rosemary, for example, is a tonic for both the body and the psyche, strengthening the will and the self and improving our sense of inner unity.

The sketch by Walter Roggenkamp attempts to illustrate the nature of the labiate plant family. Permission to use this drawing and several others from Wilhelm Pelikan's wonderful book *Man and Medicinal Plants* was kindly given to us by Editions Triades. The artist does not seek to precisely reproduce the outer appearance of the plant, but reveals in his own way what nature has concealed: the powers common to all the labiates which are manifested in the diversity and wealth of this exceptional family of aromatic plants with its approximately 3000 medicinal species forming essential oils.

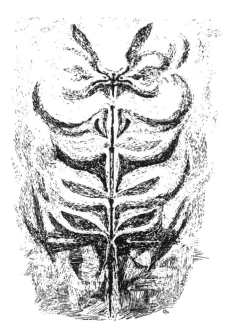

The nature of the entire family of labiates (sketch by Walter Roggenkamp)
—with friendly permission of Editions Triades.

17

A further relationship between plants and their influence on human beings was discovered by the German biologist Dr. Dietrich Gümbel. According to his research, the effects of essential oils on the skin obey certain rules which can be illustrated as follows:

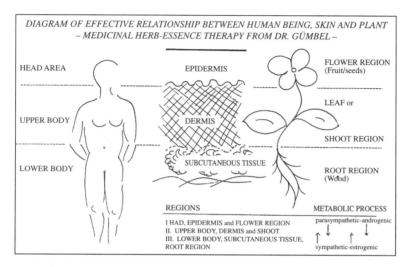

DIAGRAM OF EFFECTIVE RELATIONSHIP BETWEEN HUMAN BEING, SKIN AND PLANT – MEDICINAL HERB-ESSENCE THERAPY FROM DR. GÜMBEL –

Printed from: Gümbel, "Gesunde Haut mit Heilkräuter-Essenzen", with friendly permission from the Karl F. Haug Verlag, Heidelberg

It would certainly be beneficial to consider these interesting observations on the selective effects of essential oils on various skin layers and body zones for both therapeutic measures and personal hygiene.

From Plant Alchemy to Aromatherapy

When you look more closely at plants, you will become aware of what wonderful laboratories they are. Like all living organisms, a plant feeds on the elements of its environment. It uses the water in the soil, including the mineral salts which it contains, the air with its carbon dioxide, and above all, the sun's energy. Thanks to photosynthesis, the plant can capture the energy of sunlight and, with the help of chlorophyll, transform it into physiologically usable energy.

Photosynthesis permits the plants to breathe and transforms basic simple substances, which are poor in energy, into more complex ones which have a higher energy content. From carbohydrates (sugars), the products of photosynthesis, plants manufacture supporting substances which determine their external form. The plants also use carbohydrates to form heterosides, organic acids and fatty acids, from which lipids and oils are produced. In addition, plants also synthesize the terpenes and aromatic compounds from which essential oils are produced. These are extremely complex oils since they consist of 50 to 250 different substances.

Finally, with the help of enzymes, plants also produce amino acids and proteins, alkaloids, hormones and so forth. Plants are therefore a very rich source of many substances indispensable to life, as well as those which are beneficial in the treatment of human disorders: sugars, starches, lipids, proteins, vitamins, mineral salts, trace elements, essential oils, antibiotics, hormones, lactic acids and so forth.

Plants benefit from the great variety found in nature. The organic substances which they contain are present in physiological doses, which is why they are more easily assimilable and more potent than chemical substances manufactured with the same constitution: their own chemical constituents have been naturally synthesized and balanced by the environment of the plants and the biological transmutations which occur inside of them.

One example of this is that scurvy cannot be cured with synthetic vitamin C (commonly called antiscorbutic), even when taken in large quantities. However, it is easily healed with natural vitamin C extracted from lemons or cabbage. Drug manufacturers are well aware of this fact. Their vitamin C tablets contain 1000 mg of synthetic vitamin C and must be taken once or twice daily. Yet, the daily requirement for adults is only 75 mg, which a single small orange provides!

As a link in the natural chain of life, it is generally easier for human beings to make use of products extracted from nature itself than those which are artificial. As Professor Lucienne Béranger-Beauquesne points out: "All biosynthetic processes in the plant or animal kingdom take place by using the same enzymes and have identical or similar receptors; synthetically-produced substances, however, are generally foreign to the human organism."

Much research work has been dedicated to the diverse effects of the essential oils in general and to the specific oils in particular. (See chapters IV, VII and the Bibliography.) The medicinal substances contained in essential oils have effects that go beyond controlling the symptoms displayed by an illness: they stimulate the body's natural defences and strengthen the entire organism. When properly used, essential oils are capable of positively influencing the terrain, which means rendering innocuous the temporary or permanent influences which weaken an organ or a function and make it more vulnerable to illness. It is therefore important to have a good knowledge of plants and essential oils in order to make informed choices from this large pharmacy of nature. However, people knowledgeable about working with medicinal plants and essential oils are unanimous about one point in particular: despite their complex composition, the whole plant or the entire essential oil is more effective and successful in restoring the inner balance than any of its individual parts. This is confirmed by Dr. P. Belaiche in his important treatise on phytotherapy and aromatherapy: "The plant in its totality offers a great many different possibilities for potential effects. This explains why a more complete and extensive effect is achieved on what is called the patient's terrain."

If the plants or the essential oils are high quality, if a precise indication has been diagnosed, and if they are taken in correct doses, no undesirable side-effects are to be expected.

At the heart of aromatherapy is the use of essential oils or aromatic plant essences. This type of healing art is based on many thousands of years of experience, as well as on extensive modern research work carried out over several decades in many different places. It has good prospects of becoming a form of therapy for the future: as an alternative to chemotherapy and hope for the many afflicted who orthodox medicine cannot heal.

"Every afflicted person has his own physician within himself. The best we can do is to give this inner physician the opportunity to act."

(Dr. Albert Schweitzer)

20

Chapter II

Taking Responsibility for Our Health

Medical Science: Wisdom or Technology?

The medical science of earlier ages was founded on wisdom, knowledge, and experience. Today it primarily is a sum of highly specialized skills. We have apparently forgotten the foundation for understanding illness, which is the process of health, the foundation for our life. We must first know what enhances our harmony or causes disharmony within us. In order to achieve healing or at least an improvement of the disturbed equilibrium, one of the following approaches can be selected:

- Specialized allopathic medicine;
- Terrain therapies, which means comprehensive approaches of orthodox medicine such as homeopathy, phytotherapy, aromatherapy, oligotherapy, and oriental medicine and so forth;
- Psychosomatic or holistic medicine, which seeks to treat the person as a whole;
- The art of living in harmony with the laws of life.

At first glance, these four different approaches appear to run in opposite directions. But in the practice, use is often made of a number of possibilities at the same time. On the one hand, we may then have the strong, often complete dependence on the modern, excessively specialized medicine. It studies cases, symptoms and diseases, intensively applying technology and laboratory for the purpose of analyzing life processes.

Contrasting with this is the autonomy of a lifestyle which attempts to live according to sensible rules of self-awareness and environmental consciousness in order to become capable of restoring a temporarily impaired equilibrium without external help; instead, the person adheres to certain rules for living and eating

There is naturally a great difference between tablet consumption and the art of living. However, nothing prevents us from gradually approaching this art of living by avoiding medications that do more harm than good and favor those which stimulate our own powers of resistance.

Knowledge About Basic Hygiene

Selecting herbal medicine means we choose to be helped by nature, of which we are a part. It also means committing ourselves to a way of life which tends to reject reliance on orthodox medicine, particularly of the variety which emphasizes the use of chemicals. Those who would like to take their health into their own hands first of all must pay increasing attention to basic hygiene (and do this together with a possible therapy).

This type of preventive care is emphasized because many of us easily become weary of its simple daily demands. Yet, it plays a decisive role in our condition, whether we are healthy or not, and for our "terrain."

1. Breathing

It is important to learn to breathe better and more deeply by becoming aware of how our lungs receive the oxygen which fills our blood and all our cells with life. When we breathe, the air penetrates into our lungs and is distributed throughout the entire body by means of 100 m^2 of lung membranes. Approximately 5 liters of blood are regenerated every minute or so. This fact gives us an idea of how important breathing is as a function and of the significance of air quality we as the foundation for good human health.

Oxygen and the rest of the elements found in the air represent half the nutrition our bodies need. It is beneficial, for example, to do Hatha yoga breathing once or twice a day for ten minutes in a relaxed posture. First breathe the air deeply into your belly and then fill your lungs. With your shoulders raised, hold your breath for a moment and then slowly exhale, pushing the air out of your lungs first and then your belly.

"When you breathe it is your best meal," said O.M. Aivanhov. In the East, "schools of breathing" exist where many disorders are successfully treated with the aid of therapies which are principally based on breathing.

2. Food

We should eat better foods, which means learning to be sensitive to the needs of our organism and recognizing what may be damaging to it. Discovering some basic rules of nutrition means eating more fruit, raw vegetables, and whole grains; less meat, fats (particularly fried or cooked), and sugar. We must take into account the fact that fruit and raw vegetables are digested in the intestine (and must therefore be eaten at the beginning of a meal), while proteins, fresh dairy products, and oils are digested in the stomach; foods containing starches like bread and grain products are already broken down in the mouth by the effects of saliva and chewing. Sweets eaten at the end of a meal slow down digestion, causing fermentation and flatulence.

The fact that our bodies consist of 75 % acidic and 25 % alkaline elements must also be taken into consideration. In contrast, the ratio of acidic to alkaline elements in our diet is often precisely the opposite since it usually consists of:

• approx. ¾ acid from acid-forming foods such as meat, heated fats, heated dairy products, plus all of the chemically treated, industrially produced products like white flour, canned foods, etc. All sweets, all acidic fruit, except for lemons which have an alkaline effect in the stomach, are acid-forming.

• approx. ¼ alkaline-forming foods from fresh and raw vegetable, raw dairy products, some fruit, most whole grains (can possibly be enjoyed as sprouts), as well as some oleaginous produce like sesame, hazelnuts, and almonds.

Owing mainly to our Western eating habits, our bodies must constantly make considerable efforts in order to maintain the acid/alkali balance necessary for good health. It is then no wonder that perpetually ignoring this important biological law over a longer period of time leads to an acidification of the tissue for the majority of the population. This sets the stage for many of the so-called diseases caused by civilization (digestive, circulatory, and nervous disorders) and degenerative diseases (rheumatism, arthrosis, disorders of the immune system, cancer).

It should also be important to us to enjoy our food in a quiet and relaxed atmosphere or try at least to maintain our inner peace while eating.

3. Movement

More movement does not mean just becoming busier but rhythmic movement which suits our body, creating a harmony between muscle activity, breathing, and the heartbeat. Moving in harmony is learned, for example, by running, hiking, swimming, skiing, and practising yoga. Such types of movement have a revitalizing effect: breathing becomes deeper and the mind purified. This results in relaxation and better sleep.

4. Thoughts

We should rediscover the fundamentals of our life and have trust in our own inner being and nature, as well as what connects us with all creatures, the forces of nature, and the cosmos. These types of fundamental experiences help us to have positive thoughts and are an unsuspected source of energy.

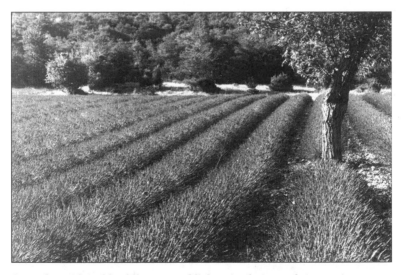

Lavender, with its blue blossoms and light, stimulating and penetrating scent, is an important medicinal plant. It is good for ailments caused by an impaired metabolism since it stimulates the respiratory, digestive, and circulatory functions, calming the nerves and heart. Lavender in baths is helpful for sciatica, gout, rheumatism, and some forms of paralysis. Lavender heals wounds, burns, and stings.

Nature as Physician

The advocates of all types of healing arts must admit that it is nature that heals. Every type of therapies or drugs can only support nature in this process.

The ability to become healthy power is within us, not outside us. This is what Pasteur meant when he said: "The microbe is nothing, the terrain is everything." Seen in this perspective, any kind of healing is self-healing. Our bodies restore their own balance. In a larger context it is the unity of body, soul, and mind that once again restores its inner harmony.

It can be dangerous to eliminate symptoms (which are an expression of our organism's will to defend itself) without giving due attention to the actual causes of an illness. Every illness is an alarm signal, which means that a person is transgressing against the fundamental laws of nature. It is not the signal that requires attention, but its cause, the fault. True healing can therefore only occur if biological laws are respected. This means that in order to make healing possible for our organism we must change our lifestyle and choose natural, non-toxic products and therapies.

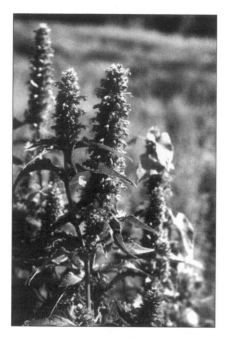

Agastache

Chapter III

Special Characteristics and Advantages of Essential Oils

Definition

Essential oils, or aromatic plant essences, are volatile, fragrant substances with an oily consistency which plants produce. They can be more or less fluid, are sometimes resinous, and often have a coloring which ranges from pale yellow to emerald green and from blue to dark brownish red. With a few exceptions, they are lighter than water and have a density between 0.75 and 0.98g/cm³. They are different from solid and liquid fatty substances because of their volatility, which increases with rising temperatures: the oily mark left by an essential oil on paper will quickly evaporate, leaving no trace. Accordingly, essential oils rapidly change from a liquid to a gaseous state; they are easily inflammable and burn with a brilliant flame. One of their physical properties is called diathermy, which means that the energy potential of an essential oil in gaseous form is increased by light passing through it since the oil retains the caloric energy of the light.

Most plants contain essential oils, but often in such minimal concentrations that either extraction would not be worth the effort or the price of the essential oil would be too high. Only the so-called aromatic plants produce essential oil in sufficient quantities. These types of plants mainly belong to the labiatae family (lavender, thyme, savory, sage, mint), the umbelliferae family (caraway, anise, fennel), the myrtaceae family (eucalyptus, cajeput, niaouli), the conifer family (pine, cedar, cypress, juniper), the rutaceae family (lemon, orange, bergamot), and the laurel family (cinnamon, borneol, sassafras). Essential oils are principally contained in the flowers and leaves of plants, but are also found in their wood, fruit and peels, bark, seeds and roots. The essential oils are formed with the help of solar energy acting on the aromatic plants' secretory cells. The plant keeps it in tiny glandular pockets which burst open, for example, when a leaf is rubbed. This is how their aromas are released. The difference between aromatic and non-aromatic plants can be determined in this simple manner.

Essential oils are soluble in alcohol, ether, and oils, but practically insoluble in water and then only dispersible with the aid of emulsifiers.

Extraction

Most essential oils are extracted from the plants by steam distillation. (It would be more correct to call the common procedure "steam passage" rather than distillation). The following factors should be observed for distillation:

A. the optimal time of harvest for the plant
B. the treatment of the plants before distillation
C. the correct distillation time in order to obtain the best yield
D. the correct pressure/temperature ratio in the distilling kettle
E. special know-how since it is sometimes advantageous for certain plants to distill them several times with rest periods in between, for example.

The essential oils of some plants, such as cloves and the peels of citrus fruit, can be extracted easily. It used to be common (and still is practiced in Sicily) to extract the essential oils of citrus fruit, for example, with a special technique: the fruit peels were scraped and the oil collected with a sponge.

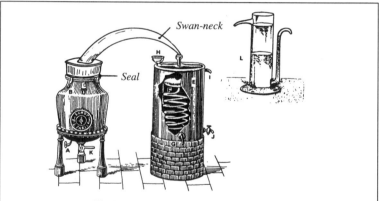

The Egrot Steam-Distillation Kettle System
A. Steam inlet B. Distillation kettle of galvanized copper for intake of plants C. Galvanized copper lid D. Swan-neck E. Cooler case of tin F. Cooling coil of galvanized copper G. Outlet for water containing essence H. Funnel I. Overflow outlet J. and K. Drainage faucets L. Florentine bottle for separation of essence from water.

Tapping is another method used on some trees, like the commiphora tree (for myrrh), the laurel of Guyana, or the camphor tree of Borneo (for borneol).

Another method is to use heat to separate various essential oils from raw resin. For example, turpentine is separated from pine resin in this manner. There are also other methods of extraction which in certain cases make it easier to obtain the essential oil or greatly increase its yield. However, this may be detrimental to the essence's quality. For instance, the plants are immersed in chemical solvents in order to obtain the volatile substances. The essential oils extracted in this manner are intimately mixed with the solvent, from which they must be separated afterwards by either fractionated distillation or some other technique. But this never shows satisfactory results: traces of solvents (hexane, acetone, methanol, isopropanol, or chloric solvents) always remain in the essential oils made in this manner .

The "enfleurage" method is similar. A fatty substance is used to absorb the essential oil, which is then separated from the substance. This method is suitable for cosmetic products since the fats loaded with essential oils can be processed into ointments, creams, and the like.

Essential oils extracted with the help of solvents are not to be used for therapeutic or hygiene purposes. Before you buy essential oils, ask your supplier about the production methods for the respective oils, particularly when they are from low-yield plants (see chapters VII, Problem of Plants Yielding Small Quantities of Essential Oil).

Concentration

The powers of aromatic plants are stored in the essential oils in a highly concentrated form. For example, when 100 kg of fresh plants are distilled they yield the following amounts of essential oil:

rose and violet	3 - 8 g
common melissa	15 - 20 g
bergamot, geranium, rosewood, thyme	100 - 300 g
wormwood, marjoram, hyssop, nutmeg, myrtle, parsley, garden sage	300 - 400 g
juniper berries, laurel, patchouli, common lavender, sassafras	1,000 - 1,200 g
cypress, eucalyptus	2,000 - 3,000 g

These high concentrations lead to the following observations:

• Essential oils are precious and must be chosen, used, and stored with care.

• For low-yield plants, the cost of extraction is very high. As a result, good quality, pure, unadulterated essential oils cannot be cheap, especially if they are of organic or wild origin. If they are sold inexpensively, it can only mean that they have been adulterated. This is a dishonorable practice, which is unfortunately much too common. Depending on the kind of substance that has been added and the intended purpose of the essential oils, it may be either merely annoying, or in some cases actually harmful and dangerous. It is therefore very important for the consumer to be informed about the quality of the essential oils purchased.

• Because of the high concentration, the essential oils must always be diluted before use. (See "How to Use Essential Oils," pg. 69 ff) Such concentration also has some advantages for practical use. Essential oils do not need much room; they can be easily transported and simple to use. They can be combined with each other in a wide variety of ways and can be made into preparations for many different purposes. They do not spoil and can be kept for 3 to 5 years if they are pure, natural, well-filtered and stored in dark glass bottles away from light and heat.

Chapter VI provides more extensive information on the consequences which high concentrations have for therapy.

Chemotypes

In order to avoid confusion, the name of an essential oil should always be derived from the botanical name of the parent plant. More and more refined therapeutic applications as well as a greater knowledge of plants have shown that, some plants belonging to the same variety, have different chemical constituents. These differences were sufficiently important to lead to the creation of "chemical races" or differing chemotypes or chemotypes. The most typical example is that of thyme (Thymus vulgaris); seven main chemotypes were recently discovered, all of which contain different substances which were present at a concentration of between 30% and 90% in each plant.

For these thymes, the chemotypes in which the following substances each dominate: cineol, geraniol, linalol, terpineol, thujanol, thymol, or carvacrol. The last two are thymol or strong thymes (also called "red thyme" by the distillers when thymol-based, and "black thyme" when carvacrol-based.) They mainly grow on the south side of chalk hills close to the Mediterranean Sea. Their leaves are grayish and the plans have quite a pungent and acrid scent and taste. These thymol-based thymes are very effective for acute infectious diseases, but they have two disadvantages:

1. They have a slightly caustic effect on the skin and are somewhat hepatotoxic (causing liver damage) when taken in large doses and over a long period of time. Pure thymol-based thymes should therefore not be used directly on the skin. This precaution should also be taken with other essential oils containing phenol, particularly those extracted from savory, wild marjoram, clove, cinnamon, nutmeg, and rosemary.
2. When taken internally, thymol-thymes should only be used for brief period of time or in very small doses. Otherwise, milder thymes should be selected.

The first fives thymes mentioned are called "mild thymes" (or yellow thymes). The geraniol-based thymes (lemon thymes) have bactericidal properties similar to the thymol-based thymes. Linalol thymes (for example, a type called "pegasus") have a milder, more subtle scent and taste. The Spanish cineol (or eucalyptol) thymes are completely non-toxic

Several other plants such as rosemary, wild marjoram, and eucalyptus contain various chemotypes. However, the non-expert should basically keep the distinction between the essential oils with either a high or low concentration of phenol in mind when using the oils. The alternative is to follow the recommendations of an aromatherapist.

In most cases, the botanical name of the plant is adequate for identification and proper use of the essential oil. For certain aromatic plants and essential oils which have a number of variations or chemotypes, it has been observed that the therapeutic indications more or less remain the same. For example, all plants belonging to the eucalyptus variety have antimicrobial and respiratory (relieving and expectorating) properties, also aiding in the healing of wounds.

Quality Features for the Consumer

The terms "pure and natural" guarantee that the essential oil has been extracted only from the plant indicated on the label and not been mixed or adulterated with other substances. This is the minimum requirement to be insisted upon by the user since there are numerous forms of adulteration, from the dilution of the essential oil to the manufacture of 100% synthetic products.

The term "organic" additionally guarantees that the oil does not contain residues of pesticides or undesirable minerals. In addition, both "organic" oils and those which have been extracted from wild plants are of better quality and possess a greater radiance. Their use is particularly recommended for aromatherapy. Because more manual activity is required to cultivate the plants, these essences are more expensive.

The specification "total" essential oil indicates that distillation has been carried out with the goal of extracting the unchanged, complete essence with all of its components. This sometimes requires a distillation period of several hours.

Terms such as "for use in food" and "for pharmaceutical purposes" are actually superfluous and add nothing to the above quality descriptions.

In conclusion, the consumer should ask for the following guarantees:

- Certification regarding parent plant (botanical name), if possible the chemotype.
- Guarantee of extraction through steam distillation at low pressure.
- Statement regarding cultivation methods like "organic" or "from wild plants."

Quality Controls at the Manufacturing Plant, Laboratory, and Pharmacy

1. Sensory tests

- The *coloring* changes with the age of the essence and its degree of oxidation, often leading to a brownish hue.
- The characteristic *odor* of each essential oil (and even of its origin,

although this can only be determined with a well-developed sense of smell).

- The *taste* is also specific to each essential oil and a good indicator. Low quality or adulterated essential oils often have an unpleasant taste, which increases in intensity with time.

2. Physical tests

- Certain common adulterations can be detected by the *test of solubility* in ethyl alcohol. Evidence may be found of blends containing turpentine, terpenes, vegetable oils, or even petroleum.
- Determining the *optical rotation* (polarization) provides indications about the purity of an essential oil.
- Its *density* to the third digit after the decimal point must be precisely established.
- The *refractive index* must be established to the third digit after the decimal point at 20°C.

3. Chemical analysis

- Tests for the *acid, ester, and hydroxyl values.*
- Tests to determine the content of *phenols, terpenes, ketones, cineols* provide information on the chemical composition of essential oil.

4. Apparative laboratory analyses

- *Spectrometry* and *spectrography* permit the exact determination of an essential oil's components.
- *Thin-layer chromatography* as well as *liquid and gas chromatography* enable the detection of even minor amounts of existing components. With these analyses it is possible to easily distinguish whether foreign substance have been added; however, they are relatively expensive tests.

5. Measurements with Vincent's bio-electronimeter

Louis Claude Vincent's work is very interesting. With his method it is not only possible to define the *quality* and *characteristics* of a fluid, but it also provides valuable information about a person's biological terrain, his equilibrium, his degree of intoxication, and his true physiological age. These measurements permit a type of assessment of the overall state of health.

Louis Claude Vincent defines his approach in these terms: "With the help of bio-electronics, it becomes clear that each living organism and each mineral solution can be precisely defined by 3 factors: its pH, rH_2, and specific resistance.

These three of these measured values are derived from the properties of water, which is the beginning of all life. There are dissociated molecules present in water to varying proportions, giving it an alkaline (OH) or an acidic (H+) character.

1. The *pH-factor* (hydrogen ion concentration) measures the number of H+ ions and thereby indicates a solution's level of acidity on a scale from 0 to 14. A pH of 7 means the solution is neutral; with a pH of less than 7, the solution is acidic; a pH of more than 7 means it is alkaline. Good quality essential oils have a pH of about 5 (maximum of 5.8) and are therefore slightly acidic.

2. The *rH_2 factor* (redox potential) measures the potential of a solution's electron transmission on a scale of 0 to 42. The neutral point is at 28. At a rH_2 of less than 28, the solution has a reducing effect and is electron-negative. A rH_2 of more than 28 means the solution is oxidizing and electron-positive. Most essential oils have a rH_2 of about 15 (maximum of 24). In accordance with this, they have a reducing effect. There are some exceptions like oleum menthae piperitae (peppermint oil), which is oxidizing.

3. The *"r" factor* (specific resistance) measures the resistance to the flow of an electrical current which a solution displays. This is measured in ohms (Û). The purer the solution, the greater the resistance with which it opposes an electrical current. Essential oils are solutions with a high level of resistance. Their "r" is greater than several thousand ohms. However, for the present, we do not wish to give precise figures since results obtained from various analyses do not agree. However, the

quality of the essential oils under analysis appears to be an important factor in the evaluation of an essential oil's quality.

For freshly distilled essential oils, these three measurements are consistent enough to attest to their quality or indicate that changes or adulterations have occurred. Experiments are currently in progress to refine these measurements to the point that they can prove whether the oils originate from the chemical or organic cultivation of aromatic plants.

Let us add a comment on what these measurements reveal about the significance of these essential oils for therapy. The acidic pH of essential oils partly explains their bactericidal properties. Acidity contributes to creating a sterile environment, whereas an alkaline pH encourages the growth of micro-organisms. In addition, a certain level of acidity is required for vitamins to become active and it helps reduce the rH-value of the blood, which should normally be around 22. If the rH_2 of the blood reaches 28, the neutral point, it can no longer fix oxygen. This condition heightens the risk of thrombosis and asthma attacks.

The reducing abilities of essential oils also explains how they help our body fight viruses and degenerative ailments. The exceptionally high specific resistance of essential oils is particularly interesting with respect to its effect upon infections and intoxications.

Risks and Toxicity of Essential Oils

Concentrated essential oils are not the topic of this book. They must by all means be diluted before use and applied in the appropriate dosage.

*"Everything is poisonous, and nothing is without poison.
The dose alone prevents something from being a poison."*
                                                              (Paracelsus)

The appropriate dosage is to be derived from the average dose, taking into consideration the particular sensitivity of each individual. Even the best things can have a harmful effect if taken in quantities which are too large or at the wrong time. Honey, for example, is a wonderful food and medicine when consumed in small quantities between meals. However, when eaten after a large meal it not only disturbs digestion, but causes particularly annoying fermentation.

Aromatherapy is a natural healing method which is remarkably effective and free of risks when used in the proper manner. The aromatherapist can adjust the doses with great precision to treat mild cases, as well as serious and acute cases require quick and effective intervention. As a result, aromatherapy can also have undesirable and even dangerous effects when used improperly. Dr. Valnet writes: "Precisely because of its influence, every effective therapy can also become harmful to the same degree as it is effective. For this reason, we should not limit ourselves to simplistic generalizations: "Everything natural is good, and everything chemical is bad." There are also poisonous plants and nontoxic, useful pharmaceutical products.

Some essential oils may be toxic when taken in very large doses or over a long period of time. This applies mainly to those which contain ketones (camphor, thuyone, and carvone) Like wormwood, hyssop, common sage, thuja, anise, fennel, caraway, rosemary, and mint. All of these may cause nervous disorders and convulsions in sensitive people , and even trigger epileptic fits in persons prone to them.

However, the incidents reported by various doctors have always been caused by doses which were too large or treatment continued over a period of time which was too long (several months or even years). Moreover, in most cases the people involved were predisposed to nervous disorders. The quality of the essential oils in question proved to be very dubious in a number of cases. If you comply with the recommended dosage and attentively observe the resulting effects, there is virtually no risk of damage caused by essential oils.

Techniques and Tools of Modern Steam Distillation

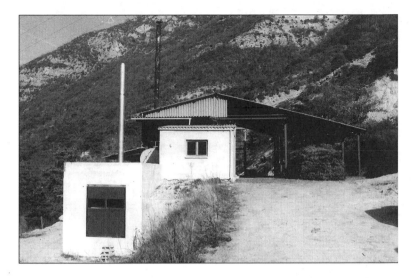

Pictures of the Sanoflore Distillery are provided here as an illustration. This very modern distillation installation is made completely of rust-free steel. It was developed by Rodolphe Balz after many years of research throughout Europe and the world. From this research, a prototype emerged which is a synthesis of the traditional knowledge about the art of distillation which has been handed down and the scientific knowledge of modern technology. The result is a distillation facility which has a variety of applications (because it can be used for the distillation of more than one-hundred different types of aromatic plants, trees, fruits, etc.). This process uses mountain spring water, which is changed to steam under low pressure and conducted through the plants to be distilled from several directions.

The three main methods can therefore be performed with the same apparatus. On the one hand, it is possible to choose the best method for optimal quality and the greatest possible yield of essential oil; research and comparisons that have scientific validity can be conducted on the other hand.

37

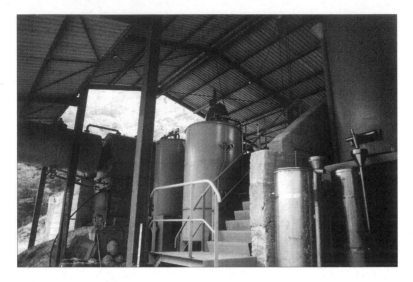

a) *The classic method:* Steam enters from below into the container (still), rises up through the plants, and leaves the container at the top through the "headpiece" or "swan-neck" (because of its shape, this is the name given to the lid that directs the steam into the cooling coils in the traditional distillation apparatus).

This method developed from the ancient observation that steam rises in the air. The fact that this apparently doesn't operate in the same way with plants gave rise to the research on the second method.

b) *Hydrodiffusion* (named after its patent application in Switzerland) turns around the direction of the steam's flow and allows it to pass through the plants from top to bottom in the container. The yield of essential oils from certain plants is increased as a result, promoting the extraction of the complete essential oil which includes its the heavier parts as well. This method also allows an economical use of energy since distillation occurs at an even lower pressure than with the classic method.

This technique is based on the observation that steam cools a bit when coming in contact with the plant, forming thicker "droplets" and charging itself with the plant's water-soluble characteristics. It follows the law of gravity, which must be compensated for by increasing the pressure in the first method.

c) *Cohobation*: This method was applied by the alchemists and the spagyric art of healing according to Paracelsus. When the hydrolate (aromatic flower water) has been separated from the essential oil, it can be reused as it leaves the essence bottle. This can be done by vaporizing it once again, and then having it pass through the plant a second time or even more frequently with the classic or hydrodiffusion method.

The hydrolate is charged with the water-soluble characteristics with every round, becoming hyper-concentrated in the process. With every round through the essence bottle, the essential oil that has been "carried along" is further decanted.

In this manner, the cohobation method allows an increased amount of essential-oil extraction from aromatic plants that contain a minimum of it, such as meadowsweet, St. John's Wort, and melissa, all of which have practically no yield when distilled. Even with the cohobation method, seven tons of fresh flowering plants are necessary in order to extract one kilogram of essential oil. This gives us an idea of how valuable the essential oils from these important healing plants are and why melissa has the well-deserved nickname of "herb of the century."

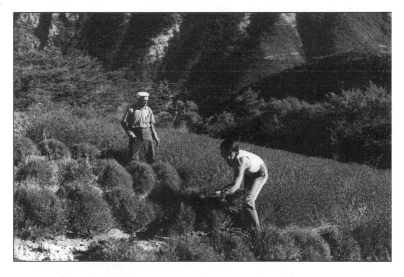

Lavender harvest in the fields near the "Sanoflore" distillery.

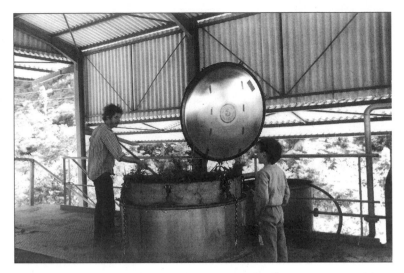

Rodolphe Balz has just filled a medium-capacity distillation container with lemon balm.

Making steam from spring water is done in three different steam kettles, depending on the special requirements of the particular plant being distilled.

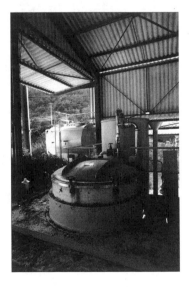

Once the plants are pressed together well, the container (shown here with 5,000 liters) is hermetically sealed with eight "security vents."

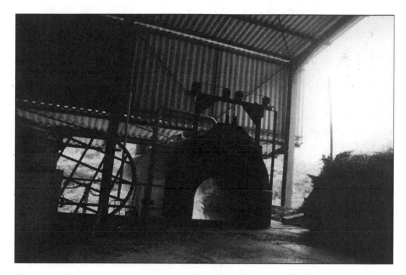

Steam kettles run on a straw or wood basis make it possible for a part of the "straw" (residue) from plant distillation to burn; however, it requires around two hours of heating before enough steam is created to begin with the distillation.

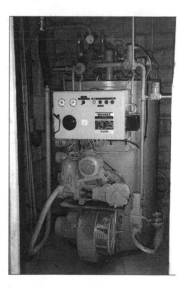

The small gas steam kettle (vaporax) works ingeniously well and allows immediate steam output.

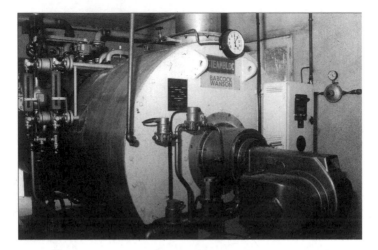

The large gas steam kettle with considerable supplies permits substantial amounts to flow through it during distillation over a longer period of time (as in the required 25-hour distillation time for parsley seeds).

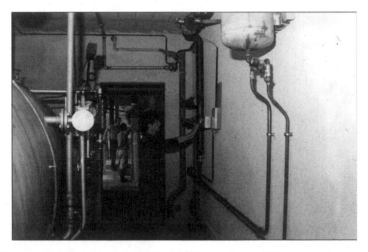

The steam kettle and its installation facilities make possible to vary the regulating and controlling of pressure, flow-through amount, temperature, degree of steam moisture, etc.

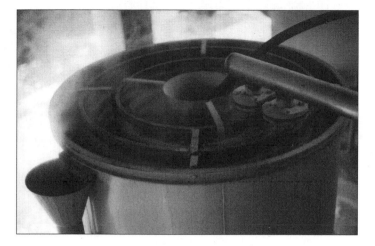

The steam flows through the plants and draws out the essential oils. At the container's outlet it cools and condenses in the double or triple cooling coil that leads down to the cooling kettle. This cooling kettle is filled with water, which is continually replaced with cold water.

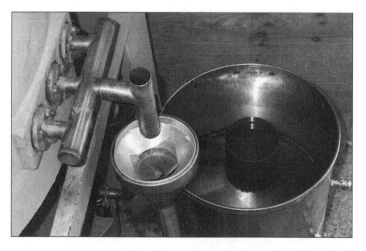

The essence bottle (or Florentine bottle) under the cooling kettle receives the condensation which is composed of the essential oil and the steam. Along its path, this gets transformed into flower water or aromatic hydrolate by charging itself with all water-soluble plant material. In this manner, the hydrolate absorbs a portion of the aromatic and medicinal properties of the plants.

The essential oil is the lightest ingredient of the condensate. It floats on top of the hydrolate in the case of most plants and then gradually forms a deposit. It is collected separately at the upper edge of the essence bottle.

Some essential oils, such as that of spice cloves, are heavier than water. A specially constructed essence bottle is required for this purpose. Others, like the essential oil of parsley seeds, contain a portion of essential oil which is heavier than water and a part which is lighter.

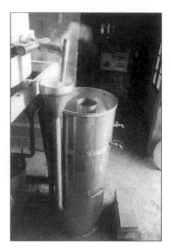

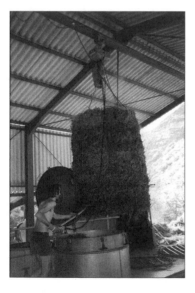

The basket with the "candle" of the distilled plant is removed from the distillation container by a helper.

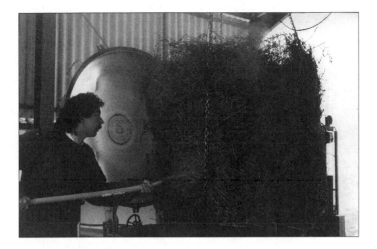

Franck, the Sanoflore distillery's responsible director decides whether the "straw" (residue) from the distilled plants will go to the compost or be used as heating material for the steam kettle.

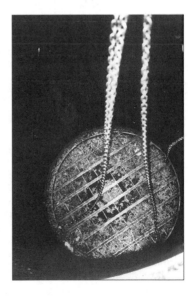

The empty "basket" or grate is lowered back to the floor of the distillation container to pick up the next load.

An experimental distillation facility, constructed according to the model of the large one, but in the ratio 1:100 (50 liters = 5,000 liters), makes it possible to run test distillations using all three of the methods cited. In this manner, a new plant can be checked to estimate the potential yield or to determine the optimal stage for cutting (the harvest) in order to obtain the best quantitative and qualitative essential oil. Eric, the director responsible for the Sanoflore research farm, regulates the last settings before distillation. This trial installation was completed using medical-laboratory glass distillation parts, with which a few hundred grams of plants can be distilled.

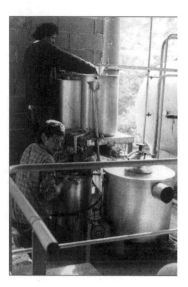

Chemistry and Medical Properties of Essential Oils

Modern aromatherapy, and especially the doctors and researchers involved, have developed two apparently contradictory procedures which actually complement each other:

The analytical procedure consists of substantiating the primary effectiveness of the essential oils on the basis of their various biochemical components, determining in particular the relationship of structure and effect through the chemical family. In the hydroxl group (hydrogen-oxygen or OH group) with C9 and C10 structure, for example, the analysis demonstrates that the mechanism of the aromatic phenols, which have proved to be a strong agent against infections, is to directly effect the pathogens to render them innocuous and indirectly effect the terrain or immune system by strengthening and stimulating it.

This procedure has led to interesting and more precise data for the therapy which is based on chemotypes and related to the quantitatively or qualitatively dominating molecule of a certain essential oil.

The analytic procedure, represented by numerous university professors and in particular by P. Franchomme and D. Pénoel, is capable of accurately analyzing the chemical family and examining the properties of each molecule in detail through test tube tests.

The synthetic procedure proceeds from the discovery that the analytic results from the test tube test "in vitro" often differ from the clinical events observed on the living object "in vivo." This difference appears to be due to the complex structure of the essential oils, the varying molecules of which develop compensatory or synergistic mechanisms which are influenced by the terrain or immune system of the patient. For example, the isolated thymol with concentrations in a magnitude of 1 : 1,000,000 cannot heal a purulent inflammation of the bladder, while the complete essential oil of (red) thyme proves to be successful. The pure eucalyptol molecule also does not achieve the goal for certain respiratory-tract diseases, while the essential oil made from eucalyptus globulus promotes complete healing. This procedure has been advocated by doctors like Valnet, Lapraz, Duraffourd, Belaiche, who based a portion of their work on the results of the aromatogram which emphasizes the significance of the patient's terrain or immune system in relationship to the choice of essential oils.

A good understanding of both of these procedures opens up the "middle way," which takes into consideration the holistic approach necessary for human beings and uses the essential oils like precious remedies for health. It is useful to know these essential oils in detail.

This means that *one* of the elements influencing the choice of one essential oil or the other for the treatment for an illness is related to the oil's chemical composition. The knowledge of essential oils according to chemotypes can be decisive for the effectiveness of a treatment. This is particularly true when the precisely determined botanical species offers significant chemical variables: Thymus vulgaris, Rosmarinus officinalis, Melaleuca quinquenervia (niaouli), and so forth.

In the following section is a summary of the most important chemical families from which the essential oil are composed. Included are their characteristic therapeutic properties.

Main Components of Essential Oils

Biochemical Elements and Therapeutic Properties

The active ingredients in essential oils are terpene-hydrocarbons with the general formula $C_{10}H_{16}$ and their derivatives, created through oxidation. When strong oxidation occurs, terpenoids are the result.

1. Terpene, Terpene-hydrocarbons or Sesquiterpene

These are quite prevalent in a large number of essential oils. Composed of carbon and hydrogen, the two main groups follow the long carbon chain; the monterpene $C_{10}+10$.

Examples of terpenes: Pinene, camphene, phellandrene, limonene, silvistrene, terpinolene, myrcene, fenchene, and others.

Plants that are rich in these components: Many of the conifers, certain umbellifers and citrus fruit such as cypress, fir, pine, eucalyptus, coriander, lemon, cumin, carrot, rosemary, tea tree.

Effects and Therapeutic properties: General strengthening agent and stimulant, antiseptic for the air (the same thing achieved naturally in coniferous forests through constant diffusion of terpenes). The limonene lessens the effect of skin irritation caused by the citral (for this reason the effect of the whole lemon's essential oil is four times less aggressive than the essential oil of the lemon without terpene content). Hormone-like characteristics: Certain conifers and their resin oil, the Scotch pine and the black spruce for example, have a stimulating effect on the connection between the pituitary gland and the suprarenal gland cortex.

Side effects: Irritation in higher dosages; revulsive effect on the skin. In case of skin irritation, use a plant oil which quickly mitigates this effect. The essential oil from turpentine and juniper branches irritates the kidneys; these essential oils should only be used internally for a brief period as part of a healing treatments or in a weaker dosage.

Special comments: Terpenes build the carbon framework of essential oils. These molecules can be saturated, unsaturated, or polyunsaturated and are more or less complex in their structure. They don't crystallize naturally, although as hydrocarbons they polymerize through oxidation. For this reason it is important to protect essential oils from air, light, and heat to preserve them. Terpenes are easily ionized to positive. Following the dislocation of an electron (spatial distribution), the "electron cloud" is attracted to the carbon nucleus, resulting in an "electrically positive" periphery.

2. Sesquiterpene C_{15}-H_{25}; Diterpene C_{20} and Triterpene

These are rare.

Examples of terpenes: Cadinene, selinene, beta-caryophyllene, humulene, cedrene, chamazulene, farnesene, puberulene, germacrene, guajene, etc.

Plants rich in these components: Galingale, celery, cloves, juniper, cedar, true chamomile, yarrow, hops, origanum.

Effects and Therapeutic properties: General strengthening agent and stimulant, antiseptic for the air. Anti-inflammatory, with properties that work on the immune system of the polyunsaturated sesquiterpenes such as chamazulene, puberulene, germacrene. The terpenes of the green cypress connect their anti-inflammatory effect with lowering the content of gama-globulin and d-alpha globulin.

Side effects: Irritation in higher dosages.

Special remarks: Transcutaneous application is an interesting method of administration: 20% essential oil is mixed with plant oil and massaged into the skin along the spine.

3. Aromatic Phenols

Examples of terpenes: Caravacrol, eugenol, thymol, guaiacol.

Plants that are rich in these components: Essential oils which have a large content of phenolene: origanum, thyme, cloves, cinnamon, gujac, savory, etc. Essential oils which have a lesser phenolene content: rosemary, mints, anise, fennel, dill, sassafras.

Effects and Therapeutic properties: As strengthening agent with an antiseptic, anti-infectious, bacteriostatic, and germicidal effect, phenols are the "spearhead" of the anti-infectious effectiveness of essential oils. They act directly on the germ (bacteria, virus, fungus), rendering it innocuous. They stimulate the immune system (greatly increasing the alpha-globulin). Phenols, through their stimulating properties, evoke general activity of a "hyper" nature (hyperthermic, hypertone); generally stimulating for the nervous system, circulation, liver and digestion, etc.

Side effects: Irritating for the skin and toxic for the liver in higher doses. Its mechanism of action with its broad spectrum and great efficiency requires precise attention to dosage and certain precautionary measures in application.

Special comments: For internal use: correct dilution for short-term use (one to three weeks) or in weaker dosage for longer treatment periods. For external use: dilute with about 5% plant oil, avoid mucous membranes and eye area.

4. Aromatic Alcohols

Example of terpenes: Terpineol, citronellol, thuja oil, cedrol, etc. Can be differentiated: Monoterpene alcohol: borneol, menthol, linaloe oil, geraniol, nerol, etc. Diterpene alcohol: salviol, sclareol, etc. Sesquiterpene alcohol: carotol, santalol, viridiflorol, etc.

Plants that are rich in these components: Lemongrass, lemon, marjoram, thyme, lavender, orange, rosemary, ravensara, mints, rose geranium, sage off., muscat sage, carrot, sandalwood, melaleuca, and others.

Effects and Therapeutic properties: General stimulant, stimulates immune resistance, bacteriostatic, germicidal, and balancing. Individual effect in terrain treatment: hormone regulation, similar structure as human sex steroids. Viridiflorol is similar to estrogen and strengthens veins.

Side effects: Soothing. Neither internally or externally toxic.

Special comments: These alcohols are not toxic with normal dosages (experiments with mice: with dose of 1 ml/kg of thymus vulgaris, thuja oil 4-chemotype, no mortality after fourteen days). Their remarkable and diverse properties make them effective medications and supportive remedies for health in children and adults.

5. Aromatic Oxides

These originate from phenol-methyl-ether compounds.

Examples of terpenes: 1-8-cineole (the most frequently occurring oxide in essential oils), linalool oxide, menthofurane, ascaridol, bisabol oxide, piperiton oxide, safrol.

Plants that are rich in these components: Eucalyptus, mints, cardamom, spike lavender, niaouli, cajeput, rosemary off., lavender-leafed garden sage.

Effects and Therapeutic properties: Strengthening for the air passages, expectorant, sedative, for allergies and asthma: linalool oxide (climbing hyssop, inula graveolens); anti-spasmodic, analgesic, for bones and joints, parasiticide (lice, crabs), fungicide (boldo).

Side effects: Beneficial for external application. Certain types can be irritating in strong dosages used internally (anaesthetic).

Special comments: Safrol, suspected of having a carcinogenic effect on human beings (sale is prohibited therefore in Switzerland, for example), is toxic and causes mutation (carcinomas) of the liver in rats. This occurs in connection with hydroxlmetabolites and epoxysafrol. It is, however, shown that this carcinogenic effect does not apply to humans. In fact, the liver-enzyme system in humans prevents the occurrence of epoxysafrol or first changes it to dihydroxysafrol and then to trihydroxysafrol, which does not cause mutations (according to P. Franchomme, D. Pénoel).

6. Aromatic Ether

Examples of terpenes: Methyl chavicol, methyl salicylate, methyl cinnamate, methyl eugenol, transanethol, methyl ether (myrtenocarvacrol, thymol).

Plants that are rich in these components: Basil, tarragon, wintergreen, cypress, anis-ravensara, cloves, bay laurel.

Effects and Therapeutic properties: Balancing, anti-spasmodic, sedative, for conditions of anxiety and depression.

Side effects: Beneficial for external use. Can be irritating and anesthetizing when used internally in high dosages.

7. Terpene Esters and Terpeneless Esters

Esters frequently "surpass" the alcohol present in essential oils. They are electro-negative and create positively-charged currents.

Examples of terpenes: Linalyl acetate, bornyl acetate, cinnamic acetate, terpenyl acetate, neryl acetate, myrtenyl acetate, menthyl acetate, eugenyl acetate.

Plants that are rich in these components: Lavender, bergamot, rosemary, pine, cinnamon, eucalyptus, cypress, birch, sassafras, helichrysum italium, myrtle, peppermint, cloves.

Effects and Therapeutic properties: Calming and relieving, balancing, anti-spasmodic, and analgesic (effects the muscles and nervous system), anti-inflammatory.

Side effects: Beneficial, non-toxic.

Special comments: The combination of the three forms of use (by way of olfactory nerves, transcutaneous—on the solar plexus—and oral) should be taken into account in the case of esters in the same way as with alcohol.

8. Aromatic and Terpene Aldehydes

Examples of terpenes: benzaldehyde, cuminaldehyde, anisaldehyde, cinnamaldehyde, citrole, citronellol, vanillin, myrtenol, neral, citral.

Plants that are rich in these components: Bay laurel, patchouli, cumin, anise, rosemary, cinnamon, lemon, lemongrass, melissa, vanilla, verbena, benzoin, fennel, cat mint, bergamot, citronella grass, eucalyptus citriodora.

Effects and Therapeutic properties: Sedative, local anti-inflammatory, strong effect against infection as a result of aromatic aldehyde (especially cinnamaldehyde), antiseptic for the air, effect on the immune system, dissolves stones (bladder and kidney stones), antiviral (herpes).

Side effects: Non-toxic; however, it is possible to determine tearing and coughing, as well as irritation of the mucous membranes and the skin, because of the cinnamaldehyde from the peel of Ceylon cinnamon.

Special comments: Risks are greatly decreased by using the correct dosage internally and being careful with essential oils containing citralene and cinnamon.

9. Aromatic Ketones (Ketoxide-Effect)

An athylene compound binds oxygen to carbon. There are several types of ketones: monotones and diketones, terpene ketones, and cyclic and acrylic ketones.

Examples of terpenes: Carvone, thujone, camphone, verbenone, cryptone, pinocamphone, borneone, fenchone.

Plants that are rich in these components: Dill, caraway, mint, thuja, sage off., eucalyptus, Japanese camphor, cinnamon, verbena, rosemary, hyssop, white fir, helichrysum, common mugwort, artemisia, lavender.

Effects and Therapeutic properties: Expectorant, slightly anaesthetic, regenerative, heals wounds of the skin and mucous membranes, anti-hemorrhagic, antiviral, bactericide, fungicide, and parasiticide (vermifugal, vermicidal).

Side effects: Neurotoxic effect of "epilepsy" type in higher doses; brings on menstruation with risk of abortive properties.

Special comments: General stimulant in weaker doses (1-2 drops undiluted essential oil), especially for the nervous system; with higher doses the effect reverses and ultimately becomes toxic. Cumulative risk, even with weaker doses, when used over a longer period of time. Preferred use on the skin or through the air for children and pregnant women.

10. Aromatic, Aliphatic Acids Containing Terpenes

The acids are strongly oxidized substances, relatively water soluble and react to alcohol with the formation of esters. They are generally present in small amounts, except in resin oils. They have a strong effect.

Examples of terpenes: Benzoic acid, cuminic acid, phenylacetic acid, salicylic acid, geraniol acid, isovaleric acid, lauric acid, myristic acid, camphone acid, citronellol acid.

Plants that are rich in these components: Ylang-ylang, orange (blossoms), cumin, birch, wintergreen, rose geranium, spiraea, valerian, laurel, nutmeg, juniper, and others.

Effects and Therapeutic properties: Calming, anti-inflammatory, lowers blood pressure, hypothermic, stimulates cell growth.

Side effects: non-toxic.

Special comments: The acids are relatively water-soluble, which is why a great portion of them reappear in the hydrolate.

11. Sesquiterpene-Lactones

These are present in small quantities in essential oils (0-3%).

Examples of terpenes: Alantolactone (= helenine), alpha-santonine, iridone.

Effects and Therapeutic properties: Expectorant, anti-infectious, vermifugal, stimulates the liver (bitter constituent), anti-spasmodic, anti-inflammatory, blood coagulant, hypothermic.

Side effects: Neurotoxic effect with medium or strong dosage; causes allergic reactions when applied to the skin.

Special comments: Considering the small amount of lactonene present in essential oils, the toxic effect is weak or non-existent when the preparation is taken properly diluted and in normal doses. Properly dilute when using externally.

12. Coumarins

Examples of terpenes: Angelicine, bergaptene, xanthyletine, limetine, visnadine, herniarine, scopoletine.

Plants that are rich in these components: Angelica, bergamot, lemon, common mugwort, parsley, limette, ammi visnaga, lavender, melissa, and others.

Effects and Therapeutic properties: Blood coagulant, sedative, decreases reflective irritation, anti-spasmodic, lowers blood pressure, hypothermic.

Side effects: Photosensitizes when applied to the skin.

Special comments: Furocoumarin and pyrocoumarin have a photo-sensitizing effect when a person enters the sun in the hours following internal or external use (wine-red spots occur as a result). This effect becomes stronger during simultaneous perspiration.

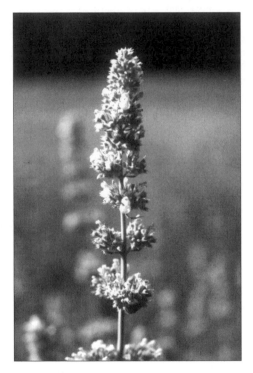

Melissa

Chapter IV

General Properties of Essential Oils

Some Examples of Their Disinfectant Properties

It is difficult to present detailed information on the many properties of essential oils here. For this reason, we would like to mention some aspects of their surprising antiseptic and bactericidal properties, as related mainly by Dr. J. Valnet in his book on aromatherapy.

* The essential oil of cinnamon kills the typhus bacillus at a dilution of 1:300.
* The essential oil of chamomile has considerable bacteriostatic properties due to one of its constituents, azulene. Azulene is effective at a dilution of 1:2000 against the staphylococcus aureus, the hemolytic-beta streptococcus (causing scarlet fever and acute rheumatic fever), and the proteus vulgaris. Infected wounds have been healed using a dilution of 1:17,000 (up to 1:180,000).
* The essential oil of *lemon* is also endowed with remarkable properties. The work of Morel and Rochais has proved that the vapors of lemon essential oil neutralize meningococcus, typhus bacillus, pneumococcus, staphylococcus aureus, and hemolytic-beta streptococcus within a short time. It also kills typhus bacillus and staphylococcus in 5 minutes and diphtheria bacillus within 20 minutes. A few drops of lemon juice on oysters eliminates 92% of their germs in 15 minutes (C. Richet).

With respect to the above experiments, it should be noted that the antiseptic and bactericidal properties of essential oils are different and more potent when administered "in vivo" than in the test tube "in vitro." Cavel's experiments established the minimal dose of essential oil needed per cubic centimeter to hinder the growth of microbial germs in one liter of bouillon contaminated with water from a septic tank:

0.7 ml essential oil of thyme
1.0 ml essential oil of origanum

1.6 ml essential oil of verbena
1.7 ml essential oil of Chinese cinnamon
1.8 ml essential oil of rose

In order to achieve the same effect, 5.6 ml of phenol (a common hospital disinfectant) is required. Yet, phenol is in 25th place on the test list—behind many essential oils.

In order to kill bacteria in the air, Professor Griffon carried out the following experiment: mixtures of various essential oils were sprayed as mists in a room. The development capacity of the germs suspended in the air was studied before and after spraying. Before the test there were 210 germs, of which 12 were molds and 8 staphylococci. Within 30 minutes, the essential oils had destroyed all the molds and staphylococci, leaving only 8 of the other germs alive. The use of essential-oil sprays for prophylactic purposes in hospital rooms, working and living spaces has therefore been demonstrated. These results are extremely interesting in light of the fact that only four or five germs per cubic meter exist in any forest, about 20,000 per cubic meter in a city apartment, and several million in a department store. There were some 5 million germs per square meter on a work table and approx. 9 million per square meter on carpeting in a busy passageway.

Summary of the General Properties of Essential Oils

Essential oils are among the most complex substances synthesized by aromatic plants at the peak of their development. They contain a large number of medicinal substances, which is why the spectrum of their therapeutic applications is so broad.

A brief summary of the properties of essential oils is given below. This list is not exhaustive and will expand with the results of further research and new applications.

1. Physical properties
Essential oils are extraordinarily diffuse and penetrating, most likely owing to their high degree of vibratory capacity. They emit electromagnetic rays of varying wavelengths and can counterbalance the vibratory

deficiencies possibly occurring in certain organs and the nervous system (see Laville and Lakhowsky's work).
- *Recommended essential oils*: all of them.

2. Properties Which Disinfect and Strengthen the Immune System

- Antiseptic (inhibiting the growth of microbes and killing them). *Recommended essential oils*: most.
- Bacteriostatic and bactericidal (inhibiting the spread of bacteria and killing them). *Recommended essential oils*: most.
- Antibiotic. *Recommended essential oils*: particularly yew, burdock, cypress, honeysuckle, but also sage, lavender, rosemary, parsley (through modification of the terrain).
- Antiviral. Viruses causing shingles, herpes, influenza, and colds can be successfully treated with certain essential oils. *Recommended essential oils*: especially lemon, pine, lavender, thyme, rosemary, sage, niaouli.
- Antimycotical and fungicidal (inhibiting the growth of fungi and molds and destroying them). *Recommended essential oils*: especially cedar, laurel, lavender, savory, mustard, thyme, tea tree.
- Wound-healing (also for burns). *Recommended essential oils*: especially chamomile, lemon, eucalyptus, geranium, lavender, myrrh, niaouli, rosemary, sage.

3. Properties which stimulate and promote functional equilibrium

- Detoxifying and antitoxic properties, notably through stimulating the organs responsible for eliminating waste products: skin, kidneys, lungs, intestines, liver, and pancreas. Because of these cleansing properties, useful against rheumatism and stones, and to help purify the blood.
Recommended essential oils: a large number, including garlic, lemon, chamomile, cypress, eucalyptus, juniper, origanum, rosemary, sage, thyme, beach pine.

- Positive effect on vessels: Some essential oils strengthen the walls of the blood vessels and stimulate blood circulation, both in the veins and capillaries, ensuring better nutrition, oxygenation, and elimination. *Recommended essential oils*: especially garlic, anise, Chinese anise, birch, cinnamon, caraway, carrot, celery, lemon, cypress, mint, nutmeg, neroli, onion, origanum, rosemary, sage, thyme.

- Heart regulatory property (low and high blood pressure). *Recommended essential oils*: see Therapeutic Index.
- Digestant properties: Essential oils promote intestinal activity, stimulate the functions of the liver and gallbladder, and are anti-flatulent. *Recommended essential oils*: especially garlic, onion, anise, carrot, lemon, fennel, juniper, rosemary, thyme.
- Catalytic and remineralizing effect by providing the cells with vitamins, trace elements, rare metals and thereby promoting metabolism and cell reproduction. *Recommended essential oils*: particularly carrot, lemon, sage.
- Protecting the cells and stimulating the body's defence mechanisms by aiding in the production of leucocytes (white blood corpuscles whose function is to intercept and destroy pathogenic agents which enter the body). *Recommended essential oils*: especially chamomile, lemon, thyme.

4. Strengthening and harmonizing properties affecting the biological field, particularly by regulating the neuro-endocrine functions on which both metabolism and all vital functions depend.

- Bio-energetic charging of the nervous system through nerve endings in the nose, tongue, and skin.
- Balancing effect on the autonomous nervous system through stimulation or calming of the sympathetic and parasympathetic nervous system. *Recommended essential oils*: see therapeutic index.
- Balancing effect on the endocrine system with the help of phytohormones (plant hormones) with a long stability. "They do not act as a substitute for deficient glands, but strengthen them. This is a stimulating physiological therapy." (Dr. J. Valnet) According to need, this therapy can either stimulate or slow down a gland's activity, thereby promoting a state of hormonal balance. *Recommended essential oils*: see therapeutic index.
- Anti-degenerative property, as a result of activating various stimulating and balancing properties. Research on their effects on tumors and cancer has shown encouraging results. *Recommended essential oils*: particularly boxwood, cardamom, cypress, honeysuckle, tarragon, juniper, lovage, pennyroyal, curled mint, neroli, parsley, balsam fir, rose, wild thyme, sage, thuja especially (as well as mistletoe, used in anthroposophic medicine).

5. Psychosomatic effect and influence on the central nervous system

Research in this field is difficult to conduct. Yet, clinical tests and daily living tell us that taking certain essential oils (such as mandarin, chamomile, thyme, sage, orange, lemongrass, neroli, marjoram, basil, tarragon, melissa, lavender) have an effect on the our moods, as well as our physical and mental well-being. They have a calming effect on anxious and sleepless people, are strengthening for the week and depressed, and relax those who are nervous, agitated, stressed, and irritable.

Certain essential oils stimulate intellectual and spiritual abilities. These are used in the spiritual realm in order to awaken centers of higher consciousness. This is why nectar and ambrosia were considered the food of the gods in ancient times, and even today in the Orient some sannyasi rub sandalwood on the point of their third eye.

In recent time, there has been a further development of medicine in two different directions. Fifty years ago, almost all therapies were "natural," yet there has been an increasing tendency toward specialization in the direction of technology and chemistry.

This tendency reached its peak in the development of synthetic medications, which selectively treat only one particular aspect or a symptom of an illness. Everything, including the human being, is broken into smaller and smaller units for the purpose of a more thorough understanding.

On the other side, there is an increasing awareness that research can only achieve its goal when the human being is considered as an integral unity, as was done in earlier times. The result has been a consciousness of so-called natural therapies, with an increasing emphasis on the global, psychosomatic, and holistic approaches. These rediscovered old methods of healing are natural in the sense that they attempt to comprehend each individual within his own specific nature and personal environment, challenging him to take an active, autonomous role in the preservation of his own health.

Both good health and illness result from an individual's lifestyle. This is perhaps the most important perception which has led to a change of attitude. From this perspective, each of us can contribute to our own preventive care, understand our own state of health and diseases, and initiate our own healing process. This means once again accepting individual responsibility since 50 years of high-technology medicine have turned human beings into passive study objects for the specialists and their medical institutions.

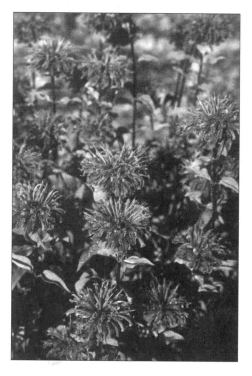

Golden melissa (Monarda didyma) was distilled in experiments and yielded very little essential oil.

Chapter V

Self-Treatment and Its Limitations

Self-Treatment

Self-treatment is highly controversial and also existent in the allopathic field: certain pharmacies are starting to resemble supermarkets. On the other hand, a constantly increasing number of people are disappointed by orthodox medicine and seek more autonomy with respect to their health. Compared with the hermetic nature of allopathy, natural therapies have the advantage of being more accessible and making the relationships between the causes of a disease, medication, and patient more understandable.

s

We can sum up our own standpoint with regards to self-treatment as follows: healthy common sense and information on the one hand and prudence and reasonable experimentation on the other. An ancient Greek proverb says: "Although we sometimes fall while learning to walk, walking is not prohibited." It is important for each of us to know the elementary rules and laws which serve to maintain our health and equilibrium, and anyone preferring to use a natural therapy in the case of health problems should have access to the appropriate information.

The neurobiologist Henri Laborit has drawn the following conclusions from his observations: When a person is urgently challenged to act because his body or environment requires it, but does not do so, this lack of response will sooner or later lead to a pathological reaction. This can be expressed on the psychological or physical level; endocrine changes result in the release of corticoids, and these in turn show a reaction in the immune system. Seen in this manner, the decision to take responsibility for one's own health-care involves the an individual's entire being and is already the first step towards healing. In the practice, sensible self-treatment requires adequate knowledge in the following three areas:
* health disorders and their symptoms
* diagnosis and causes of changes in terrain
* the remedies: (in this case, essential oils)

A correct diagnosis is of primary importance. In case of doubt or chronic symptoms, it is advisable to consult a doctor or naturopath. When using essential oils, it is important to follow the rules of use and the doses recommended in the following chapters or those prescribed by a therapist. For further information, the books about aromatherapy in the bibliography may be helpful.

The Terrain and the Aromatogram

1. The Terrain

Interest in the terrain has always played a prominent role in the history of medicine. From Hippocrates' description of the four main temperaments through Paracelsus' research work and the development of homeopathy by Hahnemann and bacteriology by Pasteur, people have always tried to understand the various states of equilibrium and regulating mechanisms of the human organism.

The comparison with the function of soil in agriculture can be used for us to understand the following section. The composition and structure of the soil are important for the development of the plants. It promotes the successful growth of some plant species and inhibits that of others. An imbalance of the soil composition encourages the growth of certain "weeds," which represent a compensatory attempt to restore the soil's equilibrium; for organic cultivation, it is a test plant. Plants grown in poorly balanced soil are weaker and more sensitive to various diseases and parasitic attacks.

In an similar manner, in human medicine an attempt is made at understanding the imbalance which has made an illness or infection possible by studying the terrain. This is the origin of Pasteur's remark: "The microbe is nothing, the terrain is everything." In modern phytoaromatherapy, various researchers have contributed to the expansion of our knowledge in this area (see bibliography).

Within the scope of this book we can only present a brief survey of this topic, but its aim is to encourage all those interested in their health to acquire information directly from the practitioners and researchers. However, you must be prepared to invest a certain amount of time when becoming involved with this branch of the healing arts. Considerable research is often necessary in order to work out an effective therapy. Progress in the understanding of this method requires detailed observations of oneself, as well as reading for continued learning and individual research in the corresponding area. Yet, our health is certainly worth the effort..

For the phytoaromatherapist, the terrain (which is also called the neuroendocrine terrain) consists of three main regulative systems:

1. **The central nervous system** is the seat of consciousness, shaped by an individual's character. It governs the neuro-vegetative system, but is also influenced by it in turn.

2. **The autonomic nervous system** regulates the automatic vital functions which are unconscious under ordinary circumstances: breathing, digestion, blood circulation and the cardiac system, etc. In order to fulfil its regulative task, this system is composed of two complementary systems:
    *   the sympathetic nervous system, which speeds up the vital functions
    *   the parasympathetic nervous system, which slows down the vital functions.
    There are four possibilities which can result from this:
    *   The sympathetic system is either speeded up or slowed down
    *   The parasympathetic system is either speeded up or slowed down.

Four types of patients can be defined in accordance with the way in which these systems function. There are four groups of essential oils which correspond to these types of patients (see Therapeutic Index).

3. **The endocrine system** consists of all the incretory glands and their hormones. These are the epiphysis, hypothalamus, anterior and posterior pituitaries, thyroid gland, thymus gland, parathyroid gland, suprarenal cortex and suprarenal medulla, pancreas, and genital glands (ovaries and testes). The pituitary gland, or master gland, stimulates or slows down most other endocrine glands. The hormones secreted by the endocrine glands and released into the blood regulate a great many specific functions. The hormonal system regulates all the major metabolic processes and is therefore the basis for our physiological, physical, and psychological reactions. Phytoaromatherapy uses plants and essential oils which balance, stimulate, or relax certain hormonal activities. (Some examples are given in the therapeutic index.)

Terrain therapy's complexity and intricacy becomes evident in the opportunity it provides for influencing all three regulative systems. However, there is a simple analytical technique which makes it possible to determine the essential oil needed for a certain patient: the aromatogram. At the same time, a fundamental clarification of the terrain conditions should not be forgotten.

2. The Aromatogram

Just as the antibiogram which tests the efficacy of antibiotics, the aromatogram tests the inhibitory properties of essential oils when in contact with pathogenic germs. This technique consists of testing a series of essential oils on isolated microbe samples taken from a patient. Each type of germ is separately inoculated on a solid culture in Petri dishes. Small paper disks impregnated with different essential oils are placed on the surface of the culture. Then it is incubated. After about 24 hours, the germs on the culture surface have grown and developed into a bacteria strain. The inhibitory effect of the essential oils is assessed by measuring the diameter of the germ-free zone, indicating the degree of the germ's sensitivity to specific essential oils. The measurements are given in crosses on a scale of 0 to 3. This laboratory test is reliable and can be reproduced on the condition that the same essential oils (not only the same varieties but also of the same origin) are used.

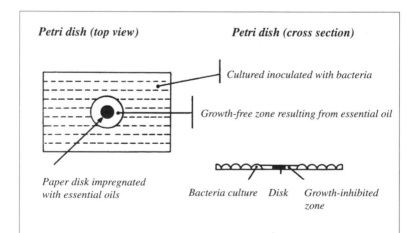

Petri dish (top view)   *Petri dish (cross section)*

Cultured inoculated with bacteria

Growth-free zone resulting from essential oil

Paper disk impregnated
with essential oils

Bacteria culture   Disk   Growth-inhibited
zone

Information on the effects of essential oils on specific germs is interesting, but it is not the most important thing revealed by the aromatogram. In the course of repeated experiments it became obvious that essential oils known for their highly disinfectant properties do not always stand out in the aromatogram. This was the case even when the illness at first seemed to be a purely infectious process. Why didn't the aromatogram emphasize those essential oils for which much research work and many published studies have established bactericidal and antibiotic properties?

The answer to this question is found in a completely new aspect of the aromatogram. The essential oils shown to be most effective by the aromatogram can be called terrain essences because they primarily have a balancing effect on the (for example, diabetic, arthritic, or neurohormonal) terrain; their secondary disinfectant and antibiotic effect is created by drainage and the restoration of the terrain's balance. It is as if the essential oil in this test first effected the carrier taken from the patient (like a smear, sputum, blood, or urine), which reveals various kinds of imbalance in the individual's physiological terrain, and that the essential oil's disinfecting properties are only revealed once the terrain has been restored.

It is therefore possible that the aromatogram recommends essential oils which do not seem to fit the symptoms, but which then prove to be an effective tool (as described above): an example of this could be restoring a pre-diabetic terrain and at the same time healing an infection with the essential oils of fennel and juniper, whose effect is hardly disinfecting.

The aromatogram permits a refining of the diagnosis while providing a better understanding of how essential oils work. It can help recognize and prevent the spread of pathogenic germs and the occurrence of resistant varieties.

Selecting Essential Oils According to Their Main and Secondary Properties

The following approach combines drainage aromatherapy with what Dr. Carillon calls symptomatic aromatherapy and attempts to tailor the treatment to the individual case. The third guiding principle of phytoaromatherapy is terrain treatment, described in the previous chapter.

All essential oils have one, two, or three main properties and several secondary ones. These various properties form a whole and work together in therapy. When a mixture of two or three essential oils is chosen for a treatment, these elements should be taken into account. We recommend the following procedure:

1. First think about your illness and try to define it as well as possible. Then consider your other potential weakness points by visualizing the various functions of your body: breathing, heart and circulation, digestion, liver, intestines, nervous system and sleep disorders, kidneys and bladder, skin, symptoms of rheumatism, and so forth.

2. Make a list of all the main symptoms (or diseases) and write down all the recommended essential oils next to them.

3. If possible, then select the essential oils common to each list. The different symptoms usually have a general relationship to each other and express deeper dysfunctions. Choosing two or three essential oils which cover these diverse symptoms increases the chances of overcoming the apparent disorder and contributes to restoring the balance of the entire terrain.

Here is an example to explain this method: A patient suffers mainly from rheumatism. By thinking about his general condition, he realizes that he is prone to high blood pressure and has liver problems from time to time. We note these three symptoms and list the therapeutically effective essential oils for each of them:

Rheumatism	High blood pressure	Liver
Birch	Carrot	Anise
Borneol	Garlic	Birch
Cajeput	*Juniper*	Boldo
Chamomile	*Lavender*	Carrot
Cypress	*Lemon*	Chamomile
Eucalyptus	Marjoram	Fennel
Juniper	Ylang-Ylang	*Juniper*
Lavender		*Lavender*
Lemon		*Lemon*
Niaouli		Peppermint
Origanum		Rosemary
Pine		Sage
Rosemary		Thyme
Sage		
Sassafras		
Tarragon		
Thyme		
Wild Thyme		
Wintergreen		

We find three essential oils (juniper, lavender, and lemon) which are in all three lists and suited for the totality of the symptoms. They can be used to make a suitable preparation for the patient's personal needs. The advantages of this simple method are obvious: it is possible to combine the essences into a mixture with an increased and more comprehensive effect. This helps avoid mistakes which may result because of the secondary properties of the essential oils. Our example illustrates this problem because if rosemary or thyme (both excellent for rheumatism and the liver) had been selected, problems related to blood pressure might have occurred after a while since these two essences can increase blood pressure.

People suffering from blood-pressure problems must take precautions when selecting essential oils by consulting the therapeutic index regarding effects on high or low blood pressure. Each time we choose one or more essential oils for the treatment of both minor and more serious disorders, it is important to take all of our weak points into account. If you want to treat bronchitis or migraine, for example, be sure to take into account a tendency toward nervousness, digestive disorders, constipation, liver complaints, etc. The therapeutic index should be consulted under the appropriate headings.

Length of Treatment

The average length of self-treatment should be between two weeks and two months in order to avoid the danger of negatively influencing the terrain as a result of an improperly selected essential oil or one which has been taken over an excessive period of time. For acute, benign, and familiar complaints, treatment must be continued for one week following the first signs of improvement, and then gradually phased out. For health cures or the treatment of chronic disorders like rheumatic complaints, never continue the treatment for more than two or three months. Afterwards, take a break from the treatment for an equal length of time. A new treatment with essential oils that have a complementary effect can then be initiated, if necessary.

Chapter VI

How to Use Essential Oils

It is important to observe the following basic rules when using essential oils in order to avoid any unpleasant side-effects:

1. Essential oils are highly concentrated substances which must always be diluted in a proper base before internal or external use. The few exceptions to this rule will explained in the following.

2. Essential oils have an oily consistency and do not mix in water or any water-based solutions. A natural emulsifier must therefore be used, which promotes a very fine distribution of the essential oil in water and contributes to the formation of an emulsion. According to the type of application, the following emulsifiers and diluents will work: "Disper," an emulsifier made from plant cells, 70% to 95% alcohol, vegetable oils, honey, yogurt, and so forth.

3. Essential oils must never be allowed contact with the eyes because this may cause severe irritation. Be careful not to touch your eyes after putting essential oil on your fingers. Be especially careful when treating children. Essential oils can cause painful irritations of the eye's conjunctiva. Ears are less sensitive in this respect. However, only the essential oils of fine lavender and eucalyptus radiata may be applied in concentrated or slightly diluted form for ear infections. No other essential oil should be introduced into the ears, except when this is expressly advised by the aromatherapist.

4. Read chapters V and VI carefully for instructions on the basic rules to follow for the preparation, dosage, and administration of essential oils.

5. Notes on abbreviations and measurement units:

   1 ml = 1 milliliter = 1 ccm = 1 cm^3
   1 g = 1 gram
   1 dr = 1 drop
   For water, 1 ml = 1 g

For essential oils, 1 ml is somewhat less than 1 G. According to the type of essential oil, 25 to 35 drops are in 1 ml, with about 35 drops in very volatile oils and about 25 drops in less volatile oils. The values vary according to the type of essential oil, the temperature, and naturally also the type of dropper cap which is used. Some essential oils are very viscous and will not readily pass through a dropper cap (vetiver, sandalwood). Others extracted from oleoresins look more like a balm or solid (balsam of Peru, guaiacwood, borneol).

Internal Uses

1. Oral Use
Taking essential oils by way of mouth is the quickest and most effective method, but also the one which requires the most caution. You should in no way exceed the doses prescribed by the aromatherapist or advised in this chapter.

2. Individual responsiveness
Each individual has his or her own level of sensitivity and responsiveness. The treatment should always start with small doses, which can then be increased up to the average dose, if necessary.

3. Selection of essential oils
All essential oils combine a number of therapeutic virtues. It is important to choose those so that the greatest number of their properties match our health disorders and weakness. Use two or three essential oils which will act in synergy (combining them to enhance and support each other's effects). For example, for an influenza infection, mix the essential oils of lemon, eucalyptus, and thyme; for digestive disorders and nervous dyspepsia, use the essential oils of basil, caraway, and savory.

4. Preparation and doses for oral use
This is the most efficient way of preparing essential oils:

1. Choose one, two, or three of the listed essential oils according to the symptoms.
2. Fill a dropper bottle to
   a) 1/10 of its volume with the selected essential oil(s)

b) 9/10 of its volume with an emulsifier ("Disper," pure 95% alcohol, or possibly grapeseed oil)
c) Shake well in order to obtain a good mixture and emulsify the contents.

According to the seriousness of the complaint, the patient should take 8 to 15 drops of this mixture in a glass of water or some herb tea. This should be done two, three, or four times a day. It is best to start with 8 drops and gradually increase the dose according to what effect it has on you. Especially sensitive people, should start the treatment with an even smaller dose of 4 or 6 drops.

Similarly, the doses can be smaller when taken on an empty stomach after waking up in the morning, which usually produces a stronger effect. People with sensitive taste buds may find the drops of diluted essential oils in water too strong. This is mainly the case with elderly people and children. In these situations as well, the doses may be smaller if the complaint is not serious. If it is, the drops can be mixed in fruit juices, vegetable juices, or herb teas (verbena, anise).

Another simple method for mixing the drops of essential oils is the use of a dropper. Here is an example for three different bottle sizes: You have chosen a preparation of four essential oils to treat a common flu without complications: lavender, thyme, cinnamon, and eucalyptus.

- **15 ml**: fill 9/10 of the bottle with "Disper" or alcohol. Add 10 drops of each essential oil (a total of 40 drops). Shake well.
- **50 ml**: fill 9/10 of the bottle with an emulsifier. Add 25 drops of each essence (a total of 100 drops). Shake well.
- **100 ml**: fill 9/10 of the bottle with an emulsifier. Add 50d drops of each essence (a total of 200 drops). Shake well. If you use only one or two essences, always add the same overall number of drops:

- 15 ml bottle: 40 drops
- 50 ml bottle: 100 drops
- 100 ml bottle: 200 drops

Proportionally, there is a little more essential oil in the 15-ml bottle. There are two reasons for this: on the one hand, the small size of the bottle implies a brief treatment for a complaint which is acute; on the other hand, the emulsion created with such a small quantity of emulsifier is slightly less effective than for larger qualities.

Adding one or two mother tinctures
(= alcoholic plant extracts)

It is possible to add a mother tincture to the mixture, using the complementary properties of a non-aromatic plant extract. In our case of influenza, for example, we could use coltsfoot. Add 50 drops of mother tincture to the 15-ml bottle, 100 drops to the 50-ml bottle, and 200 drops to the 100-ml bottle. In all of these cases, less emulsifier should be used in order to leave some space in the bottle for the tincture.

Information on mother tinctures is available in books on phytotherapy (see Bibliography). In the therapeutic index, we have in some cases used the term "phyto" to characterize certain non-aromatic plants whose properties are complementary to those of essential oils, acting in synergy with the recommended essences.

A further possibility for taking essential oils is to mix one to three drops in a teaspoon of honey and to stir well until a whitish emulsion is obtained. Dilute this mixture in a glass of water or cup of herb tea. Likewise, you can prepare the required amount of aromatic honey in advance for use in a course of treatment by carefully counting the spoonfuls of honey and drops of essential oil to be mixed.

In urgent situations, you can mix one to three drops of essential oil in yogurt, milk, or vegetable oil; if necessary, while traveling for example, you can put a tiny amount of oil on the tongue with a finger several times and immediately drink water afterwards. (Caution! Essences are very strong.)

Avoid the common method of putting some essence on a lump of sugar. Sugar is not an emulsifier and the undiluted essential oils can cause irritation when they come in contact with the mucous lining of the stomach. In addition, the stomach's power of assimilation is greatly enhanced by using a good emulsifier to distribute the essences to a much larger contact surface.

We also do not recommend taking undiluted essential oils taken in the form of capsules or breadcrumbs, etc. If you sometimes must take them in this manner, make sure you drink glass of water immediately afterwards.

5. Children's doses

a) Do not use essential oils for infants (except a few drops in the water of a humidifier or in a vaporizer to purify the air in a room). Babies should be treated with phytotherapy. Diluted herb teas are particularly suitable: one part of tea for four to six parts of water. Homeopathy also brings good results with babies. For small children (and adults as well!), food is the basic regulative agent and "medicine." Gentle massages are also recommended for digestive complaints.

b) The correct dose for children is calculated according to body weight, based on the doe for a 60-kilogram adult. (This also applies to the administration of essential oils for animals.) Here are the guidelines for doses of essential oils, tinctures, and herb teas:

- 1 to 3 years old: ⅙ of the adult dose
- 3 to 7 years old: ¼ to ⅓ the adult dose
- 7 to 12 years old: ⅓ to ½ of the adult dose
- 12 to 18 years old: ½ to ¾ of the adult dose

6. Proper time to take essential oils

The best time of day for taking essential oils is on an empty stomach in the morning after waking up. This may be enough for a maintenance therapy or it can be supplemented by a dose in the evening before going to bed. However, avoid taking the following stimulating essential oils in the evening: cinnamon, lemon, ginger, clove, rosemary, and savory. During the day, take your drops between meals or 30 minutes before a meal, with the exception of digestant preparations which must be taken after eating. People suffering from insomnia should refrain from taking stimulating preparations in the late afternoon or evening. An alternative is use two preparations: one for the morning and one for the evening (without the stimulating essential oils).

The Various Types of External Use

Essential oils have remarkable powers of penetration, diffusion, and volatility. These properties make it possible for them to be assimilated by the respiratory tract and the lungs, as well as through the skin, which they penetrate in 20 to 80 minutes. The capillaries and blood then carry them to the organs, where they are meant to have their effect, distributing them throughout the entire body. Many naturopaths consider external use the best method of administering essential oils, whereby a pleasant experience can be combined with useful treatment. Here are some examples of external application:

1. Health and Body Care

a) Inhalation

This is a simple and efficient treatment method for colds, bronchitis, sinusitis, and so forth. Put a total of 5 to 10 drops of essence from sage, pine and lavender (2—3 drops of each) in a bowl of hot, but not boiling, water. Completely cover your head and the bowl with a towel and inhale the steam for at least 10 to 15 minutes. Repeat this two or three times a day. As mentioned previously, always take the secondary properties into account when using essential oils. In the above example, sage, lavender, and thyme should be used if you tend to suffer from nervousness or insomnia. In contrast, if you feel tired and exhausted, it is better to select stimulating essential oils like rosemary, pine, or cypress.

b) Facial sauna

This pampers the face and purifies the respiratory tract. Prepare in the same manner as for inhalation. The heat, moisture, and essential oils will act in synergy on your skin. Keep you eyes closed.

- For *oily* skin: essential oils of lemon and lavender, or mint, or sage, or carrot.
- For *dry, devitalized* skin: essential oils of rosemary and lemon, or melissa, or verbena, or origanum.
- For acne and blackheads: essential oils of lavender, cajeput, and juniper, or sage, or chamomile, or geranium.
- To *cleanse and care for your skin*, and also to prevent wrinkles: essential oils of lemon and carrot, or chamomile, or orange, or patchouli.

c) Fragrant mixtures for handkerchief or pillow

Put a few drops on a handkerchief and deeply breathe in the essential oils from time to time. Or you can put a few drops on your pillow at night if you have a cold or the flu, for example: use essential oils of eucalyptus, thyme, and lavender. For fits of coughing: anise, cypress, and valerian.

d) Compresses or facial masks

Mix half a cup of clay with an herbal tea of your choice. Let it stand for a few hours, if possible in the sunshine. Add 5 to 15 drops of the selected essentials oils, according to the treatment or care required and stir well. Apply a thin layer to the skin and leave to dry. Then wash off and apply massage oil, if desired. This is excellent for general face and skin care, as well as for the treatment of bruises and sprains. For the latter, add 30 drops of arnica tincture, 5 drops each of the essential oils of sage, juniper, and chamomile, and stir in well. Apply mixture to the area to be treated. Cover with a cloth or dressing, if necessary. Repeat 2 or 3 times a day for several days.

e) Treatment and massages with undiluted essential oils

It is sometimes possible to use some undiluted essential oil straight onto the skin. This may be helpful for wounds, eczema, certain types of cramps, headaches, neuralgia, and rheumatism. The recommended essential oils are: lavender, chamomile, sage, eucalyptus, juniper, lemon, orange, etc. Thyme, oregano, savory, cloves, and nutmeg must be avoided. They are too strong for undiluted use on the skin. To test your sensitivity, put one drop of essential oil on the inside of your wrist. If no irritation occurs within 24 hours, you will tolerate the oil.

f) To disinfect, detoxify, and promote scaring

Apply one to two drops from the essential oils of lavender, eucalyptus, or geranium directly to the wound, sting, or bite.

g) For the treatment of burns

Mix equal quantities of the essences of chamomile, lavender, lemon, eucalyptus, niaouli, sage, and juniper. Apply a few drops of this blend directly on first and second degree burns. Use several times the first day and then gradually decrease the number of applications. The pain will disappear very quickly and the skin will heal in record time.

h) Massage oil for therapy and skin care

Skin-care massage oil is made with a vegetable oil or a blend of several vegetable oils beneficial to the skin (avocado, olive, almond, sesame, and wheatgerm oils) together with 3 to 5% essential oil of your choice.

In contrast, a therapeutic massage oil contains 10 to 15% essential oil. It can be used to massage and treat a weakened or affected limb or organ. For example, if your liver feels congested, gently massage the area with a blend containing olive oil and essential oils of rosemary and lemon for ten minutes.

i) Cleansing and stimulating or calming rub

A good rub with essential oils on one area of the body or the whole body stimulates, refreshes, or calms very effectively. Dip a piece of cotton-wool in some herb tea or body lotion. Then add a few drops of lemon juice and essential oils of rosemary, pine, or lemon for a refreshing effect. Rub over the whole body and face, avoiding the eyes. For a calming effect, use essential oils of lavender and chamomile, marjoram, or melissa. This treatment will quickly take effect and can be used in combination with other types of therapy for almost any complaint.

j) Healing baths

Healing baths are an important aspect of treatment with natural cures, both in the form of complete baths or as hand and foot baths (which are simpler to use). They all have a healing effect. The nerve endings of the entire body are concentrated in the skin of the hands and feet, which is why this simple therapy is surprisingly effective. (See Reflexology).

For a complete bath, add a total of 20 to 30 drops of essential oils; use about half of this amount for hand and foot baths. Stir the water thoroughly since essential oils do not mix easily with water, or add them to a bath lotion containing an emulsifier.

k) Hair care

Add 1 to 3 drops of the following essential oils to your normal shampoo or to a mild baby shampoo as required:

- For greasy hair: cedar, lavender, lemon, pine
- For dry hair: rosemary, sweet thyme, geranium, melissa, or ylang-ylang
- For normal hair: sage, thyme
- For dandruff: lavender, cade (5%)

- For blond hair: chamomile, lemon
- In case of lice, nits, hair loss (human and animals): lavender, mint, cade oil.

l) Mosquito repellant

Fragrances that keep mosquitoes and flies at bay are citronella, lemongrass, eucalyptus, geranium, and mint. Put a little essential oil directly on the skin or mix them with 70% alcohol or olive oil, using equal quantities of each.

2. Diffusing aromatic essences

The countryside and mountainous areas, even more so, have always been places where people go to recuperate and heal their diseases. This is partly because the air quality is better there and it is easier to breathe. Aromatic plants produce their essential oils with the help of the sun's energy. The wind spreads their wonderful fragrances in all directions, creating natural aerosols with ionized oxygen. The atmosphere is cleansed and the bodies of people and animals are refreshed and revitalized. This electrically charged air, enriched with volatile aromas, has a bactericidal and stimulating effect on respiration and the entire organism.

2.1 Aerosol therapy

Aerosoltherapy uses essential oils for curative purposes. The volatile and ionizing properties of essential oils can be used in a variety of ways.

a) Vaporization

There are many ways of vaporizing plant essences. For example, a few drops can be put in a water-humidifier or vaporizer. If you do not have such a device, put a few drops on a handkerchief and wrap it loosely round a light bulb which only needs to be turn on for a few minutes a day. Or simply put a bit of essential oil on a handkerchief, pillow, or blanket.

b) Spraying

Put 5% essential oil in some water or denatured alcohol and use with a sprayer. Shake well before spraying in an upward direction. You can use the following essences, alone or in combination: eucalyptus, lavender, rosemary, sage, pine, cypress, patchouli, or lemongrass. Essential oils purify and disinfect the air. They destroy the germs of contagious diseases. In addition, they bring pleasant, natural fragrances into the house.

c) Diffusion

It is possible to purchase electrically-driven aroma diffusers which produce true aerosols without the use of heat or carrier gas. A good diffuser can vaporize essential oils as a very fine mist. This greatly multiplies the ionizing and aromatizing effect of the essential oils, which have increased powers of penetration as they pass through the skin's pores. They can reach and disinfect the most remote corners of rooms, which is why they should be used for contagions diseases and epidemics.

d) Cures with aromatized air

For 15 minutes or more a day, at least twice a day in a closed room, inhale the aromatic aerosol deeply with your nose close to the diffuser. These types of cures are not only beneficial for asthma or respiratory disorders. They have a stimulating and detoxifying effect on the entire body. This is a helpful, mild, and natural therapy which complements treatment for many acute complaints of a functional or psychosomatic nature.

2.2 Pleasant perfumes

"Perfume" is not simply understood here in its fashionable cosmetic sense. In keeping with tradition, we see the fragrances as the soul or the quintessence of plants, especially of the blossoms. Aromas and perfumes have unsuspected therapeutic, revitalizing, and rejuvenating powers.

Perfumes and aromas have been intimately associated with humanity—religious rites, healing arts, and food preparation—since the beginning. A very large book would be required to cover this subject. One example is that the many murderous epidemics which hit Europe almost systematically spared the perfumers and their workshops.

Recent research has brought to light the similarity between the essential oils' aromatic chains and the bodily fluids of human beings. Blood, Lymph, saliva, and sweat all smell good when we are healthy and fit; they have a bad odor when our health is poor. Each of us has possibly experienced this fact.

The aromatic substances of plants effect the cells in human bodily fluids and stimulate the mechanisms that restore health. This means that a smell which is agreeable to us is also beneficial and useful in therapy.

Perfumes of a natural origin and good quality can also be used as aids to health.

a) Which essential oils can be used for perfumes?

A large number of essences may be used as perfumes. Examples are: bergamot, cinnamon, cedar, lemon, citronella, cypress, elemi, incense, eucalyptus, geranium, clove, lavender, lavandin, lemongrass, mandarin, marjoram, all mints, nutmeg, palmarosa, myrrh, orange, pine, grapefruit, patchouli, rosemary, rose, rosewood, sandalwood, santolina, all sages, all thymes, vetiver, ylang-ylang, and verbena.

b) How to make your own perfume

It is quite interesting to try out different blends and with the help of our sense of smell discover which ones we find suitable and enjoyable. It is best to use pure essential oils or dilute them with at least 70% alcohol.

c) Mixture ratios for perfumes, eaux de toilette, etc.

- Eau de Cologne: 3% essential oil + 70% alcohol
- Eau de toilette: 6% essential oil + 70% alcohol
- Perfume: 20% essential oil + 90% alcohol or
                       20% essential oil + vegetable oil
                       (olive, almond, or sesame)
- After-shave lotion: Eau de toilette + a little glycerin

d) Perfume fixatives

Certain essential oils fix perfumes, which means that when added to blends in small quantities they fix the volatile substances so that their fragrances last longer. Among these are: nutmeg, clove, rosewood, sandalwood, clary sage, and vetiver.

Flavoring Baked Goods and Seasoning Foods

Certain essential oils can also be used in the kitchen, and especially for baking purposes. However, you need to be careful and keep in mind that they are very concentrated ingredients. They can be diluted in strong alcohol, oils, and fats; possible also in yogurt, cream, honey, and egg yolk (must be whisked to obtain a good mixture).

You can add 10 to 30 drops of essential oils from lemon, orange, mandarin, or grapefruit for a 2-pound piece of dough. These doses are also adequate for flavoring creams, custards, ice-cream, puddings, etc. Use only 1 to 5 drops of cinnamon, cumin, anise, fennel, or clove for every 2 pounds of such recipes.

Home-baked bread can be flavored in a healthy and pleasant manner with cumin, for example. All types of dishes can be enhanced with essences from herbs. Use 1 to 3 drops diluted in 1 or 2 teaspoonfuls of vegetable oil.

One drop of parsley essence can be added to salad dressing for a special touch. However, fresh herbs are still the best thing to use.

Two pounds of honey can be flavored with 3 to 5 drops of lavender or rosemary. Mix in well. For a "sauce au pistou", 2 to 3 drops of basil are adequate. Experiment on your own to determine what appeals to you!

Chapter VII

List of Essential Oils
and Their Properties

Problem of Plants Yielding Small Quantities
of Essential Oil

The distinction between aromatic plants (which produce essential oils) and non-aromatic ones (which do not contain any essential oils) is not a strict one. There is a category of fragrant plants which contain only tiny amounts of essential oil, but which are still interesting as medicinal plants. Distilling plants whose yield in essential oil is very low poses the problem of obtaining a quality essence with a price that is still affordable.

The most common method, which are the cheapest and most efficient, makes use of solvents. However, as we have seen, toxic residues always remain in the oil, rendering it unsuitable for aromatherapy.

Another seldom used technique is high-pressure distillation which employs a liquid gas instead of steam. It delivery a qualitatively good, but very expensive product.

A third method is available: it is called "synergetic co-distillation." This is double synergy, in both the technical and therapeutic sense. For a plant with a low yield in essential oil, it is necessary to find one or two other plants which:

- Will boost the former's yield in essential oil when distilled together
- Whose combination will create a therapeutic synergy founded on common properties.
- These properties must either strengthen the virtues of the original plant or add complementary qualities to it.

Such essential oils, extracted by synergetic combination, cannot be called pure since they are obtained by distilling two or three plants together. The additions to the low-yield plant must be mentioned clearly, either by name or in a code. Some examples of this method are:

- Sapwood of linden distilled with birch
- Melissa distilled with lemongrass
- Meadowsweet distilled with rosemary from Provence

We should be aware that seven tons of fresh melissa and 20 tons of violets are needed to obtain one liter of essential oil. This explains the expensive price of these essential oils and the great temptation to dilute or adulterate them.

Since there is a trend toward natural products, there are also certain charlatans who shamelessly sell any plant under any form to treat any complaint provided they can make money in the process.

The best protection against this kind of swindle is to use your common sense and obtain thorough and reliable information.

In the last section of this chapter there is a classification of essential oils according to the frequency of their use (from common to rare) and price (from inexpensive to expensive). This summary makes it easier to select the appropriate essential oils according to the therapeutic index in Chapter VIII.

List of Essential Oils

Legend for the plant parts used:

b	—	bark
fl	—	flowers
l	—	leaves
n	—	needles
p	—	peel
r	—	resin
r	—	root
s	—	seeds
w	—	wood
wp	—	whole plant

ACHILLEA LIGUSTICA:
Achillea ligustica AILL. (wp + fl)—Asteraceae
Properties: sedative, relaxant, anti-inflammatory, antihistamine; stimulates liver and gall; supports gall production and emptying of the gallbladder; works against colds and rheumatism.
Indications: nervousness, neurasthenia, neuralgia, inflammatory processes and allergies; liver-gallbladder insufficiency; bronchitis; rheumatism.
Main components: chamazulene, 1-8 cineole, camphor, thujone.
Contraindications, side effects: abortive effect and neurotoxin if overdose is taken internally.

AGASTACHE:
Agastache foeniculum (wp + fl)—Labiatae
Properties: anti-spasmodic, nerve-regulating, anti-inflammatory, analgesic, releases vein and prostate obstruction, anti-infection.
Indications: aerophagy, gastritis, hepatitis, stomach and intestinal cramping, spasmophilia, neurasthenia, anxiety, asthenia, congestive prostate inflammation, venous circulatory disturbance, varicose veins, polyarthritis.
Main components: methylchavicol, limonene, Beta-caryophyllene, germacrene, menthone.
Contraindications, side effects: none known at normal dosages.

ANGELICA:
Angelica archangelica L. (r)—Apiaceae/Umbelliferae
Properties: stimulates appetite and digestion, carminative, general strengthening and drainage, anti-spasmodic, febrifuge, beneficial for respiratory disorders.
Indications: flatulence, nausea, palpitations, nervousness, anxiety, exhaustion, insomnia, enterospasms, kidney inflammation, uremia, malaria, for children with nervous digestion problems.
Main components: d-alpha-phellandrene, osthenol, osthol.
Contraindications, side effects: photosensitization when used externally.

ANISE:
Pimpinella anisum L. (s)—Apiaceae/Umbelliferae
Properties: appetite stimulate, sedative, anti-spasmodic, carminative, stimulates neuro-muscular and cadiovascular systems; protects bronchial system; antiseptic as intestinal disinfectant; supports breast-milk production.

Indications: stomach pain, digestive complaints, aerophagy, flatulence, spasmodic colitis, asthma, breathing difficulties due to nervousness, pounding heart, angina pectoris, painful menstruation, menopause, rheumatic neuralgic pain, intestinal parasites.
Main components: anethol, methylchavicol, anise acid.
Contraindications, side effects: dosage must be precisely complied with for internal use by children and pregnant women.

ANISE, CHINESE:
Illicium verum Hook. (s)—Magnoliaceae
Properties: stimulates appetite, strengthens stomach, carminative; stimulating tonic; relieves coughing, expectorant; neuromuscular regulant, aphrodisiac.
Indications: loss of appetite, slow digestion, flatulence; cramping cough, bronchial asthma; sexual asthenia, menopause.
Main components: anethol, pinene, phellandrene, anisic acid.
Contraindications, side effects: mastitis. Dosage must be precisely complied with for internal use by children and pregnant women

BALSAM, CANADA:
Abies balsamifera, A. balsamea L. (r)—Coniferae
Properties: cough relief, antiseptic for bronchial passages; supports wound-healing and scar formation; uro-genital complaints.
Indications: mainly external use for complaints of the bronchial system and the urogenital system; wounds; skin parasites.
Main components: beta-pinene, camphene, limonene.
Contraindications, side effects: none known for normal doses.

BASIL:
Ocimum basilicum L. (wp)—Lamiaceae/Labiatae
Properties: soothes cramps, sedative for the nervous system; anti-inflammatory, analgesic; lowers blood congestion in the veins; protects against infections, bacterial and viral diseases.
Indications: asthenia, depression, anxiety, nervous disorders, weakness of the suprarenal cortex; aerophagy, stomach cramps; viral hepatitis; rheumatic polyarthritis.
Main components: methylchavicol, cineole, l-linalool, eugenol.
Contraindications, side effects: none known for normal doses.

BASIL, LARGE-LEAFED:
Ocimum basilicum album (wp)—Lamiaceae/Labiatae
Properties: general strengthening, restorative (digestion, liver, gallbladder, circulation, and nerves), lowers blood congestion in prostrate and uterus.
Indications: liver and gallbladder insufficiency, congestion in prostate and uterus, bladder inflammation, disturbances of heart rhythm, asthenia, psychoasthenia.
Main components: linalool, fenchol, beta-caryophyllene, methylchavicol, estragol.
Contraindications, side effects: not known for normal dosage.

BASIL, EUGENOL:
Ocimum gratissimum L., Eugenol-Chemotype (wp)—Labiatae
Properties: anti-infection, bactericide (staphylococcus aureus and albus, streptococcus-beta hemolyse, pneumococcus), anti-viral; appetite stimulant, nerve strengthening.
Indications: insufficiencies of liver and pancreas; arthrosis; bronchitis, angina; nervous disorders; intestinal parasites.
Main components: eugenol, beta-caryophyllene, beta-ocimene, alpha-terpineol.
Contraindications, side effects: caustic for the skin when used externally; liver irritation when overdose taken internally.

BAY:
Myrcia acris, Pimenta racemosa miller (l + fl)—Myrtaceae
Properties: circulatory stimulant, sedative to autonomic nervous system, antiseptic, anti-infection, bactericide, heals wounds.
Indications: bladder inflammation, urethra inflammation, leucorrhea, viral hepatitis, colitis, enterocolitis; low blood pressure, asthenia; toothache, neuralgia, rheumatic polyarthritis.
Main components: eugenol, methyleugenol, chavicol, alpha-pinene, limonene, myrcene, citrale.
Contraindications, side effects: none known at normal dosage.

BENZOIN:
Styrax benzoe Dryander (r)—Styracaceae
Properties: against bronchial disorders, disinfects, expectorant; supports scar formation; for skin ailments and facial care.
Indications: breathing difficulty, wounds, growths, frostbite, burns; skin ailments, psoriasis, eczema, acne.

Main components: coniferyl-benzoate(ester), cinnamic acid.
Contraindications, side effects: none known for normal dosage.

BERGAMOT (LIME):
Citrus aurantium L. var. bergamia (p)—Rutaceae
Properties: antiseptic, bactericide; regenerative for hypothalamus; supports scar formation; stimulates appetite, febrifuge, vermifuge; skin-browning.
Indications: intestinal infections, colic, loss of appetite, intestinal parasites; insomnia, inner nervousness; malaria; wounds, skin disorders, psoriasis.
Main components: l-linayl acetate, d-limonene, bergaptene, nerol, citrale.
Contraindications, side effects: strong photosensitizing when applied externally.

BIRCH, BLACK:
Betula lenta L. (b + w)—Betulaceae
Properties: diuretic, supports passage of uric acid and chloridene; blood purifier, against rheumatism; heals wounds and growths.
Indications: gout, uremia, inadequate urine output, kidney inflammation, edema; rheumatism, arthritis; skin rashes, abscesses, psoriasis.
Main components: methyl salizyate.
Contraindications, side effects: none known for normal dosages.

BIRCH, YELLOW:
Betula alleghaniensis S. (b)—Betulaceae
Properties: relaxes cramping, anti-inflammatory, removes fluids, stimulates the liver.
Indications: rheumatism, arthritis, tendonitis, cramps; light weakness of liver; headache.
Main components: methyyl salizylate.
Contraindications, side effects: none known for normal dosage.

BOLDO:
Peumus boldus Mol. (l)—Monimiaceae
Properties: supports the flow of bile; general strengthening; diuretic; slightly hypnotic effect.
Indications: liver and gallbladder weakness; fungus disease (Candida) of intestines and vagina.
Main components: eucalyptol, ascaridol, boldine.

Contraindications, side effects: dosage must be precisely complied with for internal use by children and pregnant women.

BORNEO CAMPHOR:
Dryobalanops camphora (r)
(Dryobalanops aromatica garden) (W)—Hypericaceae
Properties: generally strengthening effect, heart-strengthening; antiseptic for bronchial disorders, pain-reliever; aphrodisiac.
Indications: physical and sexual asthenia, depression, exhaustion; cardiac insufficiency; infectious diseases; rheumatic neuralgia.
Main components: d-borneol, alpha-pinene.
Contraindications, side effects: none known for normal dosages. Not to be confused with Japanese and Chinese camphor, which is toxic due to its ketone content.

BOXWOOD:
Buxus sempervorens (l)—Buxaceae
The essential oil is obtained by synergistic co-distillation.
Properties: blood-purifier, supports flow of bile, "anti-carcinogenic"

BUCHU:
Barosma betulina (l)—Rutaceae
Properties: diuretic, disinfects the urinary tract, against colibacteria, restorative, against bronchial illness.
Indications: influenza, bronchitis; infection of urinary tract, bladder inflammation, illness caused by colibacteria; excessively slow digestion.
Main components: d-limonene, dipentene, diphenol (buchu-camphor).
Contraindications, side effects: none known.

BUPLEURUM:
Bupuleurum fruticosum L. (wp)—Apiaceae
Properties: against infection, microbes, and bacteria, kills airborn germs; general physical and mental strengthener and stimulant.
Indications: bronchial infection, infection of the digestive system; stomach and intestinal atony, asthenia, exhaustion; disinfection of air.
Main components: limonene, beta-alpha-phellandrene, carvacrol, citronellol, bupleurol (dihydronerol).
Contraindications, side effects: none known.

CADE:
Juniperus oxycedrus L. (w)—Coniferae/Cupressaceae
Properties: for ailments of skin and scalp; against parasites.
Indications: skin ailments, skin parasites, pediculosis.
Main components: cadinene, humulene, cubenol.
Contraindications, side effects: use only externally; none known for normal dosage.

CAJEPUT:
Melaleuca cajeputi Pow. (l)—Myrtaceae
Properties: antiseptic for the intestines, the urinary tract and lungs; antiviral, against rheumatism, against acne; anti-spasmodic; lowers blood congestion in veins.
Indications: diarrhea (dysentery), intestinal parasites, bladder inflammation, urethra inflammation, kidney inflammation; bronchitis, larynx and throat inflammation, rheumatism, gout; skin ailments, wounds, acne, herpes (genital), psoriasis; leuchorrhea; stomach cramps; tooth neuralgia; painful menstruation; varicose veins, hemorrhoids; dysplasia of cervix.
Main components: 1-8-cineole, alpha-beta-pinene, limonene, beta-caryophyllene, terpineol, viridiflorol
Contraindications, side effects: none known for normal dosage.

CAJEPUT LEUCADENDRON:
Melaleuca leucadendron L. (l) Myrtaceae
Properties: anti-spasmodic, relaxant; against infection, bacteria, and parasites; lowers blood congestion in the veins.
Indications: spasmophilia, spasmic and infectious enterocolitis; amoebic dysentery, intestinal parasites; varicose veins, hemorrhoids.
Main components: methyl eugenol, eugenol, cineole, alpha-terpineol.
Contraindications, side effects: none known for normal dosages.

CALAMINT:
Calamintha nepeta Sav. ssp. nepata Brig., C. pariflora Lam., C. sylvatica Bromf. (wp + fl)—Labiatae
Properties: stimulation and strengthening of brain, respiratory tract, digestion, liver and gallbladder; against infection and fungi, expectorant; regulates thyroid gland.

Indications: asthenia; insufficiency of bronchial system, bronchitis, sinusitis; digestive complaints, liver-gallbladder insufficiency, fungal diseases (Candida-mycosis, aspergillosis), hyper-function of thyroid gland.
Main components: pugelone, l-menthone, calamenthone, l-alpha-pinene.
Contraindications, side effects: use in weak dosage for internal application; do not use for children and pregnant women.

CAMPHOR (CHINA, JAPAN):
Cinnamomum camphora L. (w)—Lauraceae
Properties: generally strengthening, stimulates heart and breathing; antiseptic, anti-infective, febrifuge, analgesic.
Indications: use only externally for asthenia, dizziness, abscess, bronchitis, pain, rheumatism, sprains.
Contraindications, side effects: has a neurotoxic, abortive effect when used internally.

CANANGA:
Cananga odorata macrophylla Lam. Baill., Hook. et Thom(Indonesia, Java) (fl)—Anonaceae
Properties: anti-spasmodic, balancing, against infection of respiratory system; general stimulant and sexual tonic.
Indications: heart stimulation, high blood pressure, tachycardia; sexual asthenia, frigidity, impotence.
Main components: linalool, cresolemethylate, farnesol, alpha-farnesene, benzyl acetate and geranyl acetate.
Contraindications, side effects: none known for normal dosages.
See also under *Ylang-Ylang*.

CARAWAY:
Carum carvi L. (s)—Umbelliferae
Properties: stomach-strengthening, stimulates appetite, supports digestion, carminative, anti-spasmodic; antiseptic, vermifuge; stimulates bile production and emptying of gallbladder; expectorant.
Indications: stomach pain, digestive complaints, lack of appetite, aerophagy, flatulence, liver-gallbladder insufficiencies; bronchitis; intestinal parasites.
Main components: carvone, carvene, carvarcol, limonene.
Contraindications, side effects: dosage must be precisely complied with for internal use by children and pregnant women.

CARDAMOM:
Elettaria caedamomum L. (l + s)—Zingiberaceae
Properties: stimulates appetite, supports digestion, diuretic, anti-spasmodic; carminative, antiseptic for the bronchial system; heart-strengthening.
Indications: stomach pain, digestive complaints; rhinitis, bronchitis; flatulence, aerophagy, spasmic colitis, intestinal parasites; cardiac insufficiency.
Main components: terpenyl acetate, cineole, lanalol, limonene.
Contraindications, side effects: none known for normal dosages.

CARROT:
Daucus carota L. (s)—Apiaceae/Umbelliferae
Properties: regenerative for the liver and gallbladder; regulates intestines, against diarrhea and putrescence; stimulant, tonic for nerves; anemia; blood purifier, promotes breast-milk production; against ulcers, rejuvenating effect on skin, against wrinkles.
Indications: liver-gallbladder complaints, high cholesterol, constipation, diarrhea; breathing complaints; asthenia; uremia, kidney inflammation; skin diseases, little broken veins, eczema, pus-infected fingers.
Main components: carotol, daucol, bisabolene, 1-carotine.
Contraindications, side effects: none known for normal dosage.

CAT MINT, WITH LEMON AROMA:
Nepeta cataria L. var. citriodora Beck (wp + fl)—Labiatae
Properties: anti-infective, against microbes, bacteria, viruses, and fungi; sedative, analgesic, anti-inflammatory; dissolves gallstones.
Indications: infection of respiratory and digestive tract, inflammatory and viral diseases, herpes; spasmophilia, anxiety, nervous depression; gallstones.
Main components: geranil, citronellol, geranial, neral, methyl chavicol, caryophyllene.
Contraindications, side effects: none known for normal dosage.

CEDAR:
Cedrus atlantica Manet. (w)—Abieacreae/Pinaceae
Properties: antiseptic for respiratory and urinary tract, also for skin; supports wound-healing; strengthens; aphrodisiac.
Indications: urethra inflammation, bladder inflammation; bronchitis; disorders of lymph system, sexual asthenia; ailments of scalp, skin diseases.

Main components: cedrol, 1-alpha-pinene, himachalene, cadinene, aliphatic aldehyde, atlantol, alpha- and beta- atlantone, formic acid.
Contraindications, side effects: dosage must be precisely complied with for internal use by children and pregnant women.

CELERY:
Apium graveolens L. (s)—Apiaceae/Umbelliferae
Properties: stimulates and strengthens, carminative; strong diuretic; blood-purifying, against rheumatism, counterirritant for ailments of the respiratory tract and liver; stimulant for gallbladder; supplies minerals; aid in weight loss; aphrodisiac.
Indications: asthenia, anxiety; flatulence, kidney insufficiency; against rheumatism; consecutive symptoms of bronchitis and liver disorders; sexual asthenia.
Main components: limonene, apigenol, beta-selinene.
Contraindications, side effects: none known for normal dosage.

CHAMOMILE, ROMAN:
Anthemis nobilis L. (fl)—Asteraceae/Compositae
Properties: important anti-inflammatory; anti-spasmodic, sedative, strong disinfectant; against anemia, stimulates leucocyte development; against rheumatism; supports menstruation; vermifuge.
Indications: spasmophilia, neurasthenia, intermittent fever, influenza, angina, anemia, rheumatism, facial neuralgia; kidney inflammation, testicle inflammation; too strong or painful menstruation, nervous amenorrhea, menopause; intestinal parasites, constipation; pus-infected fingers.
Main components: isobutyl-angelate, isobutyryl, angelica-ester, pinocarvone.
Contraindications, side effects: none known for normal dosage.

CHAMOMILE, TRUE OR GERMAN:
Matricaria Chamomilla L. (fl)—Asteraceae/Compositae
Properties: lowers fever, anti-spasmodic, analgesic, strengthens stomach, stimulates appetite; against anemia; tonic, antiseptic, promotes wound-healing and scaring.
Indications: fever, malaria, headache, dizziness, neuralgia, muscle cramping, nervousness; digestive complaints, digestive disturbances in children, stomach ulcers, anemia, depression, amenorrhea, too strong or painful menstruation (nervous causes), leucorrhea; bladder inflammation, skin ailments, wounds, ulcers, eczema, burns.

Main components: chamazulene, farnesene, bisabol-oxide, alpha-bisabolol, camphor.
Contraindications, side effects: none known for normal dosages.

CHAMOMILE, WILD MOROCCAN:
Ormenis mixta L. (fl)
Properties: anti-inflammatory and antibacterial; general tonic; wound healing.
Indications: colitis and bladder inflammation caused by colibacteria, intestinal parasites, amoebic dysentery; slight liver insufficiency, stomach atony, depression; wounds.
Main components: santolina-alcohol, alpha-terpineol, 1-8-cineole, camphor.
Contraindications, side effects: none known for normal dosage.

CINNAMON, CEYLON (BARK):
Cinnamomum zeylanicum Nees (b)—Lauraceae
Properties: stimulates heart, circulation, and respiratory tract; strengthening; carminative; anti-spasmodic, antiseptic, hemostatic; important remedy against infection, bacteria, viruses, and fungi; promotes menstruation; aphrodisiac.
Indications: circulatory disturbances, vein blockage, lung and cardiac insufficiency; physical and sexual asthenia; pyorrhea; stomach atony, digestive cramps, intestinal infections, amoebic dysentery, tropical fever, diarrhea, dysentery, spasmic bladder inflammation, ailments brought on by colibacteria, intestinal parasites; leucorrhea, amenorrhea.
Main components: cinnamaldehyde, eugenol, furfural, 1-alpha-pinene, p-cymene, 1-phellandrene, 1-linalool, amyl ketone.
Contraindications, side effects: slightly caustic on the skin, especially when the essential oil is low quality or mixed with cinnamon leaves.

CINNAMON, CEYLON (LEAF):
Cinnamomum zeylanicum Nees (l)—Lauraceae
The essential oil acquired from the leaves through distillation has certain properties which are milder than those of the oil acquired from the bark. Because of its high proportion of eugenol, it is similar to the essential oil of carnation.
Properties: antibacterial, against infection, viruses, and parasites; generally stimulating, nerve-strengthening, supports the immune system.

Indications: stomatitis, tooth neuralgia; enterocolitis, bladder inflammations, vaginitis; prostatic inflammation; intestinal worms, skin parasites; rhinopharyngitis, bronchitis, physical and sexual asthenia.

Main components: eugenol, 1-alpha-terpineol, cinnamonol, safrol.

Contraindications, side effects: caustic on the skin.

CINNAMON, CHINA OR CINNAMON CASSIA:

Cinnamomum Cassia flower (b + lf)—Lauraceae

Properties: anti-inflammatory and antibacterial, antiseptic; generally strengthening, particularly for respiratory tract and nerves; anti-coagulant, hemostatic remedy for arteries.

Indications: Pyorrhea, inflammation of gums; asthenia; preventative cardiovascular treatment.

Main components: transcinnamaldehyde, benzaldehyde, isoeugenol.

Contraindications, side effects: Slightly caustic effect on skin.

CITRONELLA GRASS:

Cymbopogon nardus L. (Ceylon)—C. citratus DC. Stapf (India)—C. winterianus Jowitt (Java) (wp)—Poaceae/Gramineae

Properties: disinfectant, anti-inflammatory, antibacterial; anti-spasmodic, analgesic; digestive tonic; vascular expansion; repels insects; deodorizes, hygienic antiseptic.

Indications: infectious and inflammatory ailments, complaints of stomach-intestinal tract, colitis; malaria; diabetes; rheumatism; vegetative dystonia.

Main components: D-citronellal, neral, 1-borneol, geraniol, nerol, methyl eugenol, sesquicitronellene.

Contraindications, side effects: none known for normal dosage.

CLOVE:

Eugenia caryophyllus Spreng (s)—Myrtaceae

Properties: strong appetite stimulant; anti-spasmodic; aphrodisiac; nerve tonic; analgesic; against fungi and parasites, strong antiseptic and bactericide, supports scar formation; for skin ailments, bronchial diseases, intestinal disturbances; lowers blood pressure; against infection in tooth area and regeneration of gums.

Indications: stomach slackness, bacterial colitis, amoebic dysentery, viral intestinal inflammation and enterospasms, viral hepatitis, malaria, shingles, viral nerve inflammation; tooth neuralgia, tooth inflammation; complaints in throat-nose-ear region; bladder inflammation, physical and

mental asthenia; rheumatic polyarthritis; eases birth; vermifuge, skin parasites and pediculosis.
Main components: eugenol, methyl eugenol, caryophylline, alpha-methyl furfurol, vanilline.
Contraindications, side effects: none known for normal dosage, irritating to the skin when used externally.

COMBAVA:
Combava hystrix DC. (p)—Rutaceae
Properties: disinfectant, germicide, supports digestion; prevents blockage in liver-gallbladder region; supports circulation, neurotonic, stimulant, a particularly stimulating sexual effect.
Indications: stomach-intestinal infections, atony and blockage of the liver, bladder and circulation; ovarian and testicle insufficiency.
Main components: beta-pinene, sabinene, beta-caryophyllene, citronellal, citrale, linalool, furocoumarin.
Contraindications, side effects: photosensitizing when used externally.

COPAIBA BALSAM:
Copaifera off. L. (r)—Fabaceae/Papilionaceae
Properties: stimulating, antiseptic disorder of respiratory and urinary tract, anti-inflammatory, supports wound healing and scar formation.
Indications: infections of bronchials and lungs, as well as urinary tract; leucorrhea, wounds, and ulcers.
Main components: caryophylloene, 1-cadinene, alpha-copaene, alpha-cubebene.
Contraindications, side effects: none known for normal dosage.

CORIANDER:
Coriander sativum L. (s)—Umbelliferae
Properties: stimulating, strengthening, stimulates appetite, carminative, promotes intestinal function; antibacterial and parasites, disinfects, analgesic.
Indications: asthenia, exhaustion; digestive complaints, aerophagy, fermentation in intestines, constipation; bladder inflammation; influenza, arthrosis.
Main components: alpha-linalool (= coriandrol), geranyl acetate, alpha-beta-pinene, gamma-terpinene.
Contraindications, side effects: none known for normal dosage.

CORKWOOD, WITH LEMON AROMA:
Litsea citrata (fl) —Lauraceae
The variety "Litsea cubeba Pers" has components, properties and indications which are very similar to Litsea citrata.
Properties: sedative, analgesic, anti-inflammatory, against infection; tonic for digestion.
Indications: insomnia, nervous depression, nervous disorders, asthenia; stomach and duodenal ulcers, inflamed colitis and enterocolitis, atonic digestion; for oral hygiene, against aphtha.
Main components: citrale, neral, geranial; limonene, myrcene, linalool.
Contraindications, side effects: none known for normal dosage.

CUBEB:
Piper cubeba L. (fruit)—Piperaceae
Properties: stimulates appetite; antiseptic for urinary infection; aphrodisiac.
Indications: enterocolitis; bladder inflammation, infection of urogenital system, leucorrhea; sexual asthenia.
Main components: D-sabinene, d-d4-carene, 1-4-cineole, cubebol, cubebine, 1-cadinene, azulene.
Contraindications, side effects: danger of diarrhea when used for long periods internally.

CUMIN:
Cuminum cyminum L. (s)—Umbelliferae
Properties: strengthens stomach, stimulates appetite, carminative, diuretic; antiseptic; analgesic; promotes menstruation and breast-milk production; relaxant for smooth (vegetative) musculature.
Indications: stomach pain, aerocoli, asthenia; hepatitis; mumps; arthritis, rheumatism; insomnia; for breast-feeding; amenorrhea; (nightly) muscle cramps.
Main components: cuminol, pinene, terpineol, beta-caryophyllene, cumin aldehyde.
Contraindications, side effects: irritation caused by intensive external application on skin.

CYPRESS, PROVENCAL OR ITALIAN:
Cupressus sempervirens L. (l + cones)—Cupressaceae
Properties: hemostatic, promotes scar formation, astringent, diuretic, sudorific, febrifuge; good cough remedy; vessel-contracting, strength-

ens veins; anti-spasmodic; balancing for nervous system; against rheumatism.

Indications: wounds; edema of lower limbs; pleurisy, tuberculosis; varicose veins, hemorrhoids; prostatic tumor, bed wetting, asthenia; rheumatism; cramped and bronchial coughing; malaria.

Main components: alpha-pinene, terpineol, cedrol, sempervirol, d-camphene, d-sylvestrene.

Contraindications, side effects: mastitis.

DILL:

Anethum graveolens L. (s)—Apiaceae/Umbelliferae

Properties: promotes digestion, strengthening and anti-spasmodic, diuretic, antiseptic, vermifuge; heals wounds.

Indications: digestive problems, liver and gallbladder insufficiencies; bronchitis; intestinal parasites; wounds.

Main components: carvone, anethol, limonene.

Contraindications, side effects: abortive and neurotoxin when dosage is exceeded for internal usage.

DOUGLAS:

see under *Fir, Douglas*.

ELDER:

Sambucus nigra (fl)—Caprifoliaceae

The essential oil is acquired through synergistic co-distillation.

Properties: sudorific, diuretic, blood purifier; effective for respiratory system and kidneys.

ELECAMPANE:

Inula helenium L. (r)—Asteraceae/Compositae

Properties: antiseptic, sedative, promotes liver activity, diuretic (elimination of urea and chlorides), anti-asthmatic, soothes coughs; digestive stimulant; promotes menstruation; vermifuge; promotes scar formation.

Indications: bronchitis, liver and gallbladder insufficiencies; gout, kidney stones; asthma, coughs; digestive problems; amenorrhea or painful menstruation; intestinal parasites.

Main components: alantolactone, alantol acid.

Contraindications, side effects: allergic reactions when used externally; comply with correct dosage for internal use.

ELEMI:
Canarium Iuzonicum Miq. (r)—Burseraceae
Properties: promotes scar formation, antiseptic; good for bronchial disorders, relaxes coughing; regulates digestion.
Indications: wounds, ulcers, varicose veins; bronchitis; digestive problems, diarrhea, enterospasms, amoebic dysentery.
Main components: elemol, elemicine, dipentene, terpineol, limonene, phellandrene.
Contraindications, side effects: none known for normal dosage.

ERIGERON, CANADIAN:
Erigeron canadensis L. (wp + fl)—Compositae
Properties: diuretic, astringent, diuretic.
Indications: rheumatism, gout, kidney inflammation, albuminurea (protein in urine), diarrhea.
Main components: citonellol, menthene, delta-limonene, delta-l-terpineol.
Contraindications, side effects: none known for normal dosages.

EUCALYPTUS CAMALDULENSIS:
Eucalyptus camaldulensis (l)—Myrtaceae
Properties: antiseptic, cough relief, neurolytic.
Indications: complaints in throat-nose-ear area, neurasthenia.
Main components: 1-8-cineole, alpha-pinene, limonene.
Contraindications, side effects: avoid internal and external use by infants and small children, with the exception of spraying in the air.

EUCALYPTUS CITRIODORA:
Eucalyptus citriodora Hook. (l)—Myrtaceae
Properties: anti-inflammatory, sedative, analgesic; against rheumatism, against infection.
Indications: arthritis, rheumatism, rheumatic polyarthritis; high blood pressure; shingles; bladder inflammation, vaginal inflammation.
Main components: citronellal, citronellol, geraniol.
Contraindications, side effects: none known for normal dosage.

EUCALYPTUS DIVES:
Eucalyptus dives Schau (l)—Myrtaceae
Properties: against infection of lungs and kidneys, against colds, expectorant; regenerating for kidneys.

Indications: complaints in throat-nose-ear area, bronchitis, angina, otitis, sinusitis; kidney inflammation, uremia; vaginitis.
Main components: piperitone, phellandrene, linalool.
Contraindications, side effects: the dosage must be complied with exactly for internal use by pregnant women.

EUCALYPTUS GLOBUS:
Eucalyptus globus Labill. (fl)—Myrtaceae
Properties: antiseptic for respiratory diseases and urinary tract infections, relieves coughing, stimulating astringent, hemostatic, promotes scar formation, analgesic; against diabetes and rheumatism; against antifungal and parasites.
Indications: complaints in throat-nose-ear area, bronchitis, sinusitis, influenza, angina, rhinopharyngitis, otitis; bladder inflammation, diseases caused by colibacteria; malaria; rheumatism; wounds, skin inflammations caused by bacteria and fungi (Candida), intestinal parasites.
Main components: 1-8-cineole, d-alpha-pinene, terpineol, isoborneol, globulol.
Contraindications, side effects: avoid internal and external use for infants and small children, with the exception of spraying in the air.

EUCALYPTUS POLYBRACTEA:
Eucalyptus polybractea Baker, cryptone-cchemotype (l)—Myrtaceae
Properties: against colds, expectorant, against infection; bacteria, virus, amoeba, and malaria pathogens; lessens blood congestion in prostate.
Indications: complaints in throat-nose-ear area; epidemics due to bacteria and viruses, amoebic enterocolitis, malaria; viral and congestive inflammation of the prostate; condyloma; rheumatic polyarthritis.
Main components: cryptone, para-zymene, cuminal, 1-8-cineole, phellandral.
Contraindications, side effects: dosage must be precisely complied with for internal use by children and pregnant women.

EUCALYPTUS RADIATA:
Eucalyptus radiata Sieb. (l)—Myrtaceae
Properties: antiseptic, relieves coughs; promotes wound healing, antibacterial and virus, anti-inflammatory; derivant for humoral terrain.
Indications: complaints in throat-nose-ear area (bronchitis, influenza, rhinopharyhngitis, sinusitis, coughing and others); leucorrhea, vaginitis; conjunctivitis; wounds, acne, skin parasites; asthenia, plethora.

Main components: 1-8-cineole, alpha-terpineol, geraniol, phellandrene, piperitone, piperitol.

Contraindications, side effects: none known for normal dosage.

EUCALYPTUS SMITHII:

Eucalyptus smithii RT Baker (l)—Myrtaceae

Properties: against infection, expectorant, against colds; stimulating; derivant, analgesic, against rheumatism.

Indications: complaints in throat-nose-ear area and uro-genital region; rheumatism; asthenia.

Main components: 1-8-cineole, alpha-pinene.

Contraindications, side effects: avoid internal and external use for infants and small children, with the exception of spraying the air.

EVERLASTING, GYMNOCEPHALUM:

Helichrysum gymnocephalum Humb. (fl)—Asteracae/Compositae

Properties: important anti-inflammatory, analgesic, sedative, antiseptic; antilithic, anti-diabeticum, stimulates the pancreas.

Indications: acute limb rheumatism; inflammation of gums; inflammation of stomach lining; headache; skin ailments, herpes, ulcers; goiter.

Main components: limonene, beta-caryophyllene, alpha-humulene, citronellal.

Contraindications, side effects: none known for normal dosage.

EVERLASTING, ITALICUM:

Helichrysum italicum (Roth) var. serotinum G. Don (fl)—Asteraceae/Compositae

Properties: anti-inflammatory for veins, anti-coagulant, hemostatic; lowers cholesterol; anti-spasmodic, expectorant, against coughing; stimulates the liver.

Indications: phlebitis, internal and external hemorrhage; for shock, little ruptured arteries, wounds, arthritis, polyarthritis, Dupuytren's contracture; complaints in throat-nose-ear area, bronchitis; liver insufficiency, headaches caused by the liver.

Main components: neryl acetate, italidion, nerol, d-alpha-pinene.

Contraindications, side effects: dosage must be precisely complied with for internal use by children and pregnant women; avoid entirely with sensitivity to ketones.

FENNEL, MILD GARDEN:
Foeniculum vulgare Miller var. dulce (s)—Apiaceae/Umbelliferae
Properties: powerful diuretic, stimulating, removes chloride organisms and promotes increased production of nitrogen in the urine; expectorant, for bronchial disorders; vermifuge, anti-fungal, carminative; stimulates bile production;, promotes menstruation; promotes breast-milk production.
Indications: atonic digestion, flatulence, constipation, stones in the urinary tract, kidney inflammation, insufficient urination, gout; amenorrhea; intestinal parasites. For external use emollient: blood effusions, slight mastitis.
Main components: anethol, d-phellandrene, delta-limonene.
Contraindications, side effects: dosage must be precisely complied with for internal use by children and pregnant women.

FENNEL, WILD:
Foeniculum vulgare Miller var. acer (wp + r)—Apiaceae/Umbelliferae
Properties: tonic for nerves and digestion, diuretic; promotes estrogen-like properties of menstruation and breast-milk production, neuromuscular antispasmodic; analgesic; stimulates bile production and drainage of gallbladder; antiseptic.
Indications: stomach pain, spasmic colitis, digestive problems, aerophagy, flatulence, constipation, uremia; amenorrhea, weak, infrequent and painful menstruation, menopausal problems; asthma; pain in lumbar region.
Main components: camphene, d-alpha-phellandrene, dipenthene, d-fenchone, anethol, methyl chavicol.
Contraindications, side effects: dosage must be precisely complied with for internal use by children and pregnant women.

FIR, DOUGLAS OR OREGON FIR:
Pseudotsuga menziesii(Mirbel)(Beissn.) Franco-P. douglasii(Lindl.) Carr.—P. canadensis B. Hooker (n)—Abietaceae/Pinaceae
Properties: antiseptic, against colds, expectorant; general stimulant; germicide for the air.
Indications: infections of respiratory tract; bronchitis, sinusitis, atony of respiratory tract and circulation; freshens and disinfects the air in rooms.
Main components: beta-alpha-pinene, terpinolene, limonene, delta-3-carene, citronellyl acetate, Borneo Camphor, geraniol, camphor.
Contraindications, side effects: none known for normal dosage. Can irritate skin or mucous membranes through undiluted use.

FIR, GIANT OR VANCOUVER FIR:

Abies grandis Dougl./lindl. (n)—Abietaceae/Pinaceae

Properties: antiseptic and soothing for respiratory tract; sedative; against rheumatism; general stimulant tonic.

Indications: bronchitis, sinusitis; bladder inflammation, urethra inflammation; rheumatism; atony, asthenia.

Main components: alpha- and beta-pinene, bornyl acetate, b-phellandrene, camphene, limonene, myrcene, alpha-cubebene, alpha-copaene.

Contraindications, side effects: none known for normal dosage. Can irritate skin or mucous membranes through undiluted use.

FIR, WHITE:

Abies alba Mill., A. pectinata DC., A. excelsa lK. (n)—Abietaceae/Pinaceae

Properties: general antiseptic, especially for respiratory tract, relieves and sooths coughs, against colds, expectorant; general stimulant tonic; against arthrosis.

Indications: bronchitis, sinusitis, colds; bladder inflammation; rheumatism, arthrosis; asthenia.

Main components: L-limonene, 1-alpha-pinene, camphene, bornyl acetate, beta-caryophyllene, myrcene, alpha-humulene, laurialdehyde.

Contraindications, side effects: none known for normal dosage. Irritates digestive organs and nerves through frequent or longer use; can irritate skin and mucous membrane through undiluted use.

GALBANUM:

Ferula galbanifera Boiss (r)—Apiaceae/Umbelliferae

Properties: wound-healing, softening, promotes scar formation, derivant, antiseptic for disorders of urinary tract; stimulates intestinal activity.

Indications: wounds, hemorrhage; infection of urinary tract.

Main components: carvone, limonene, cadinene, cadinol, alpha-beta-pinene, myrcene.

Contraindications, side effects: dosage must be precisely complied with for internal use by children and pregnant women.

GARLIC:

Allium sativum L. (clove)—Liliaceae

Properties: antiseptic, bactericide, especially by ailments of respiratory tract; circulatory disorders, diseases of urinary tract, dropsy, and overweight; derivant, increases muscle tone; lowers blood pressure; vermifuge.

Indications: infectious diseases, influenza, chronic bronchitis, tuberculosis, asthma, whooping cough, runny nose, high blood pressure, vascular cramps, varicose veins, hemorrhoids; formation of urinary stones, gout, insufficient urinary excretion, edema, intestinal parasites.

Main components: diallyl sulfide.

Contraindications, side effects: skin irritant when applied externally; comply with exact dose for internal use.

GENETIAN:

Gentiana lutea L. (r)—Gentianaceae

Properties: bitter tonic, promotes digestion, blood-purifying, antiseptic, antispasmodic; against rheumatism; balances autonomous nervous system.

Indications: loss of appetite, general exhaustion, dyspepsia, stomach and intestinal atony, liver insufficiencies, diarrhea, gout, malaria; intestinal parasites.

Main components: gentiotanic acid

Contraindications, side effects: digestive problems and vomiting with high dosages.

GERANIUM, ROSE:

Pelargonium roseum asperum Ehr. cv 'Bourbon' Ile de la Reunion (wp)—Geraniaceae

Properties: anti-spasmodic, anti-inflammatory, analgesic; astringent tonic; hemostatic; stimulates circulation; against infection and fungi; promotes wound healing and scar formation, against diabetes.

Indications: nervous colitis, anxiety, agitation; liver-pancreas insufficiency; care of skin and mucous membranes, alveolar pyorrhea (infection of gums), skin ailments, wounds, skin parasites, pregnancy stretch marks, hemorrhoids, rheumatism, facial neuralgia.

Main components: geranil, citronellol, linalool, citronellyl- and geranylformiate, isomenthone.

Contraindications, side effects: none known for normal dosage.

The rose geraniums from Africa, Madagascar and Asia, as well as the variety Pelargonium graveolens show the same properties, with just a few nuances of their own.

GINGER:
Zingiber officinalis Roscoe (r)—Zingiberaceae
Properties: stimulates digestion and respiratory organs; blood-purifier; febrifuge; analgesic; against rheumatism; aphrodisiac; against scurvy; antiseptic; good for the eyes, aromatic hydrolate (ginger water).
Indications: digestive complaints, constipation; chronic bronchitis; impotence; tooth neuralgia, rheumatism.
Main components: zingiberone, d-phellandrene, gingerol, cineole, isoborneol, citrale.
Contraindications, side effects: none known by normal dosages.

GOLDENROD:
Solidago puberula S. virga aurea DC. (wp)—Compositae
Properties: anti-inflammatory, sedative, analgesic, relaxant (heart muscle), regenerative for vascular problems; dehydrating, diuretic.
Indications: arteritis, endocarditis, pericarditis, inflammation and infection of lymphatic system, anemia, cramps, inflammation of nerves, sciatica, insomnia.
Main components: puberulene, beta-caryophyllene, alpha-humulene, germacrone, myrcene, alpha-beta-pinene, germacrene.
Contraindications, side effects: none known for normal dosage.

GOLDENROD, CANADIAN:
Solidago canadensis L. (wp)—Compositae
Properties: anti-inflammatory, nerve sedative, lowers blood pressure, diuretic, stimulates liver and bladder.
Indications: arteritis, endocarditis, pericarditis, high blood pressure, neurasthenia, spasmophilia, hepatotoxemia.
Main components: alpha-pinene, myrcene, limonene, alpha-phellandrene, bornyl acetate.
Contraindications, side effects: none known for normal dosage.

GRAPEFRUIT:
Citrus paradisii Macf., C. decumana L. (p)—Rutaceae
Properties: strengthening, promotes appetite and digestion; blood purifier, derivant for liver and kidneys; hemostatic; refreshing; weight loss (together with basil and sage).
Indications: atony of digestive organs, liver and kidneys; plethora, corpulence, cellulitis; germicide (air).

Main components: limonene, alpha-beta-pinene, citrale, citronellal, octyl aldehyde, geranil, d-cadinene, furocoumarin, bergaptene.
Contraindications, side effects: photosensitizing when externally applied.

GUAJAC:
Guajacum off. L. (w)—Zygophyllaceae
Properties: antiseptic for urinary tract; strong sweat-producer; stimulates respiratory tract; against gout.
Indications: bladder stones, uro-genital disorder (especially syphilis); lung complaints, lymph-gland swelling; skin diseases; gout, rheumatism; asthenia.
Main components: guaiacol, guaiol.
Contraindications, side effects: none known for normal dosage.

GURJUN:
Dipterocarpus turbinatus Gaertn., D. alatus Roxb. (r)—Dipterocarpaceae
Properties: antiseptic for intestines and urinary tract; anti-inflammatory, for infection; for skin diseases.
Indications: bladder inflammation, urinary tract inflammation, uro-genital complaints; inflammation of bronchial tubes and lungs, skin diseases.
Main components: caryophyllene, gurjunene, guaia azulene.
Contraindications, side effects: none known.
Hawthorne:
Crataegus oxyacantha (fl)—Rosaceae
The essential oil is acquired through synergistic co-distillation.
Properties: regulates and strengthens heart, lowers blood pressure; antispasmodic; calms the nerves, for vegetative dystonia.

HORSERADISH:
Cochlearia amoracia L. (r)—Cruciferae
Properties: stimulates appetite, against scurvy, stomach-strengthening, promotes digestion, diuretic, derivant; antibacterial; stimulates capillaries.
Indications: atony and infection of digestive organs, plethora; pneumonia, disorders of capillaries.
Main components: sulphur compounds (mustard oil), allyl-isothiocyanate.
Contraindications, side effects: use only in very diluted doses, irritates the skin; pregnant women and children should avoid use.

105

HYSSOP:
Hyssopus officinalis L. (fl)—Labiatae
Properties: respiratory-tract complaints, very effective for relief of coughs and as expectorant; anti-inflammatory, against asthma; against infections, bacteria, and viruses; strengthens stomach, promotes digestion, stimulates appetite, strengthens and stimulates nervous system, raises blood pressure; softens, promotes wound-healing and scar formation.

Indications: bronchitis, lung inflammation, sinusitis, asthma; digestive complaints, metabolizing of fat; asthenia, multiple sclerosis; wounds, scars, bruises, leprosy.

Main components: isopinocamphone, 1-pinocamphone (ketone content is higher when harvest and distillation take place later in the year = fall), alpha-and beta-pinene, cadinene, beta-caryophyllene, nerol, nerolidol.

Contraindications, side effects: dosage must be precisely complied with for internal use by children, pregnant women, and people with ketone sensitivity.

HYSSOP (chemotype 1-8-cineole):
Hyssop officinalis L. (fl)—Labiatae
Properties: against infection, microbes, and bacteria; relieves coughs, expectorant; sedative, anti-spasmodic; strengthens stomach; stimulant.
Indications: infectious or asthmatic bronchitis, sinusitis, influenza; atonic digestion and digestive complaints of nervous origin.
Main components: 1-8-cineole.
Contraindications, side effects: none known for normal dosage.

HYSSOP, CREEPING WILD:
Hyssop officinalis L. var. decumbens (fl)—Labiatae
Properties: against colds, expectorant, relieves coughs, anti-inflammatory, against asthma; strengthens and stimulates sympathetic nervous systemj; against infection and viruses; vermifuge.
Indications: bronchitis, bronchiolitis in small children, rhinopharyngitis, inflamed asthma and secretious influenza; bladder inflammation; nervous depression, anxiety; intestinal parasites (tapeworms).
Main components: translinalool oxide, limonene, alpha- and beta-pinene, myrcene, linalool, 1-8-cineole.
Contraindications, side effects: none known for normal dosage (unlike the official hyssop, creeping hyssop contains less than 1% ketones, and therefore has no ketone poisons).

106

INCENSE OR OLIBAUM:
Boswellia carterii Birdw. (r)—Burseraceae
Properties: stimulates and strengthens; promotes wound healing and scar formation; relieves coughs; promotes digestion, anti-depressive, "anti-carcinogenic."
Indications: asthenia; wounds, ulcers; bronchitis, asthma; depression, (cancer).
Main components: L-alpha-pinene, dipentene, cadinene, alpha-gurjunene, alpha-guajene, transpinocarveol, farnesol.
Contraindications, side effects: none known for normal dosage.

INULA:
Inula graveolens Desf. (wp + fl)—Asteraceae/Compositae
Properties: regulates and strengthens heart and circulatory system; anti-inflammatory, anti-spasmodic, analgesic, relieves coughs; against infection, germicide, for colds, expectorant; strong derivant.
Indications: disturbances of heart rhythm, tachycardia, inflammation of aorta and coronary vessels, high blood pressure; chronic bronchitis, rhinopharyngitis, inflamed tonsils, inflammation of trachea, cramped coughing; bladder inflammation; vaginitis; skin inflammation.
Main components: camphene, b-farnegene, Borneo Camphor, bornyl acetate, lactone.
Contraindications, side effects: none known for normal dosages.

IRIS:
Iris florentina L., Iris pallida Lamk. (r)—Iridaceae
Properties: against colds, expectorant, promotes cough relief, diuretic, blood-purifier, against rheumatism; vermifuge.
Indications: chronic and asthmatic bronchitis, asthma, sinusitis, whooping cough; rheumatism; skin diseases.
Main components: myristic acid, furfural, alpha-beta-benzal aldehyde.
Contraindications, side effects: none known.

JATAMANSI:
Nardostachys Jatamansi DC (r)—Valerianaceae
Properties: analgesic, sedative for nerves (nerve plexus), vein tonic.
Indications: spasmophilia, tachycardia, nervous disorders; varicose veins, hemorrhoids; psoriasis.
Main components: dihydroazulene, valerianol, valerianal, valeranine, nardostachone, jataminsinic acid.
Contraindications, side effects: None known.

JERUSALEM OAK SEED (GOOSEFOOT):
Chenopodium ambrosioides L. var. anthelminticum (wp)—Chenopodiaceae
Properties: strong vermifuge; tonic, stimulates appetite, carminative; sudorific; promotes menstruation.
Indications: intestinal parasites, stomach complaints, flatulence; amenorrhea.
Main components: P-cymene, limonene, delta 3-carene, ascaridol, ascaridolglycol, methyl salizylate.
Contraindications, side effects: has a neurotoxic effect, avoid use for pregnant women and small children; use internally only in very weak dosage and for a short time period.

JUNIPER:
Juniperus communis L. (berries)—Cupressaceae
Properties: stimulates metabolism, digestion and kidney functioning; diuretic, blood purifier; strengthening; against rheumatism and arthritis; helps eliminate uric acid and oxalic acid, sudorific, antiseptic, against diabetes, promotes wound healing and scar formation, slightly sleep-inducing.
Indications: gallstones, liver-pancreas insufficiency, digestive complaints, infectious enterocolitis, insufficient urination, kidney inflammation; pericarditis; rheumatism, gout, arthritis; dental neuralgia; wounds, ulcers, skin ailments, eczema, acne; leucorrhea.
Main components: terpinole-4, camholenic acid, camphene, cadinene.
Contraindications, side effects: none known for normal dosage.

JUNIPER, COMMON:
Juniperus communis L. (berries + branches)—Cupressacea
Properties: general stimulant; against rheumatism; diuretic, antiseptic; against colds, expectorant, cough relief.
Indications: rheumatism, arthritis, liver-pancreas insufficiency; gallstones, bronchitis, rhinitis.
Main components: L-terpinene, alpha-pinene, camphene, cadinene, terpenyl acetate.
Contraindications, side effects: none known for normal dosage.

JUNIPER, MOUNTAIN OR DWARF:
Juniperus communis L. var. montana (berries + branches)—Cupressaceae
Properties: stimulates digestion and stomach-intestinal tract; against infection; stimulates immune resistance; sedative, anti-inflammatory, analgesic, anti-spasamodic; regulates vegetative nervous system.

Indications: rheumatism, arthritis, sciatica; spasmic colitis and enterocolitis and related conditions caused by fermentation; neuritis; vegetative dystonia; skin ailments.

Main components: pinene, limonene, camphene, bornyl acetate, terpenyl acetate.

Contraindications, side effects: none known for normal dosage.

JUNIPER, SAVIN:

Juniperus sabina L. (l)—Cupressaceae

Properties: promotes menstruation (abortive); hemostatic; analgesic; vermifuge; tonic.

Indications: amenorrhea, uterine hemorrhage; worm ailments. Used externally for eczema, wounds, ulcers.

Main components: alpha and beta-pinene, sabinene, terpinene, cadinene, geraniol, citronellol, sabinol, (poldophyllotoxin).

Contraindications, side effects: avoid internal use, especially by children and pregnant women, or use only under medical supervision.

JUNIPER, VIRGINIA (RED CEDAR):

Juniperus virginiana L. (w)—Cupressaceae

Properties: stimulates circulation, relieves and strengthens the veins.

Indications: hemorrhoids, varicose veins, phlebitis, venous stasis.

Main components: cedrene, cedrole, cedrenene, thujopsene.

Contraindications, side effects: none known for normal dosage.

LABDANUM:

Cistus ladaniferus L. (l)—Cistaceae

Properties: against infection and viruses; hemostatic; regulates vegetative nervous system; astringent and strengthening; promotes scar formation and healing of wounds; for disorders of chest cavity.

Indications: infectious childhood diseases, viral diseases, bleeding, diseases of the auto-immune system; rheumatic polyarthritis, multiple sclerosis, vegetative dystonia; wounds, ulcers.

Main components: alpha-pinene, camphene, Borneo Camphor, labdane-8-alpha, labdaneol, acetophenone, eugenone, trimethylil 1, 5-5-cyclohexanone-6, ledol.

Contraindications, side effects: none known for normal dosage.

LANTANA, SAGE, JAMAICA MOUNTAIN:

Lantana camara L. (wp + fl)—Verbenaceae

Properties: against infection and viruses; against colds, expectorant; promotes menstruation (against tumors); remedy for wound healing and scar formation.

Indications: chronic bronchitis, influenza, asthma; aphtha, ulcerated varicose veins.

Main components: beta-caryophyllene, alpha-humulene, davanone.

Contraindications, side effects: avoid use by small children and pregnant women.

LARCH, EUROPEAN:

Larix decidua Miller L. europaea (l)—Abietaceae/Pinaceae

Properties: antiseptic and disinfectant; stimulating and relaxing for nerves; for eye ailments (hydrolate).

Indications: bronchitis, pneumonia; bone dystrophy; nervous exhaustion. According to Rudolf Steiner, effective cataracts in combination with lavender oil and pineapple juice (internal application).

Main components: alpha-pinene, limonene, alpha-terpineol, bornyl acetate.

Contraindications, side effects: none known for normal dosage.

LAUREL:

Laurus nobilis L. (l)—Lauraceae

Properties: fights infections, bacteria, viruses, fungi; against colds, expectorant, relieves coughing, sudorific, anti-spasmodic, analgesic, against rheumatism, balances the sympathetic nervous system, against ulcers.

Indications: tooth neuralgia, stomatitis, aphtha; influenza, viral hepatitis, viral nerve inflammation, malaria, mycosis; infections in nose-throat-ear region; arthritis, polyarthritis, rheumatic deformities, muscle contractions; vegetative dystonia, swelling of lymph gland; ulcers, acne, boils.

Main components: 1-8-cineole, linalool, terpenyl acetate, geraniol, alpha-pinene, sabinene, methyl ether-eugenol, alpha-phellandrene.

Contraindications, side effects: none known, except for people susceptible to skin allergies.

LAVENDERS AND LAVANDINS:
There are three types of wild Lavender:
Lavender, true
(Lavandula officinalis Chaix syn. Lavandula angustifolia Mill., Mnch.): small-leafed Lavender, wild mountain Lavender, Provence Lavender, plants from the mountains of Haute-Provence which grow at an altitude of 700 or 800 to 1800 meters; main ingredient is linalool.
Spike Lavender
(Lavandula spica L.): grows on the plateaus of France and Spain; main ingredient is 1-8-cineole.
Stoechas Lavender:
(Lavendula stoechas L.):
grows in the Mediterranean region; its main components are ketone and camphor.

Many hybrid sorts of Lavender have resulted from this basic type. All of these crosses have become known as Lavandin. Lavandin types make up 95% of the production planted in the plateau and yield two to eight times as much as true Lavender. The majority of these cultures are cloned from chosen kinds for their yield of essential oils. They are therefore infertile and cannot multiply through their seeds.

Lavender is a specific plant from the southern French Provence. Its spread to other growing areas (like Romania, the Black Sea, Tasmania) is based on cloned plants, which were removed from Provence (Dept. Drome) a few decades ago. This origin from one or two cloned French plants and their multiplication explains the typical product, which is relatively simple in its composition, yet still different than the Lavender "population" of Provence. This presents, in botanic and especially in chemical terms, an unusual variety. In fact, like every clone this breed has certain primary botanic and chemical properties. Through multiplication with plant cuttings these properties are precisely reproduced, but do not possess the broad variety of natural hybridization.

LAVENDER, TRUE OR LAVANDE FINE:
Lavandula angustifolia Miller, L. off. (fl)—Labiatae
Properties: stimulates appetite, promotes bill production as well as draining gallbladder, carminative, diuretic; stimulates nervous system, but subdues cerebro-spinal overexcitation; regulating and strengthening for heart; strongly antiseptic, promotes wound healing and scar formation, anti-inflammatory; against allergies; for ailments of respiratory tract, digestive organs, the uro-genital system; against rheumatism; against

111

migraine; lowers blood pressure; promotes menstruation; against snake bites, parasites, and insect bites; beneficial effect on the skin.

Indications: infectious skin ailments, psoriasis, wounds, skin parasites, intestinal worms; leucorrhea and spermatorrhea; nervous disorders, anxiety, psychoasthenia, insomnia; nervous palpitations, high blood pressure; cramps, insufficient urination, kidney inflammation; rheumatic neuralgia.

Main components: linalyl acetate, linalool.

Contraindications, side effects: none known for normal dosage.

Spike Lavender or Wide-Leafed Lavender:
Lavandula larifolia Med., L. spica (fl)—Labiatae

Properties: anti-spasmodic, strengthening, antiseptic, antibiotic, against infection, promotes wound healing and scar formation, analgesic: stimulates appetite, promotes bile production as well as drainage of gallbladder, carminative, diuretic; against ailments of respiratory tract; regulates heart and circulation; subdues cerebrospinal overexcitation.

Indications: coughing, bronchitis, trachea inflammation; infectious skin ailments, skin parasites, wounds, burns; nervous disorders, anxiety, insomnia, high blood pressure; rheumatism, arthritis; neuritis, neuralgia.

Main components: cineole-linelol, d-camphene, d-camphor, d-borneol.

Contraindications, side effects: none known for normal dosage.

Stoechas Lavender:
Lavendula stoechas L. (fl)—Labiatae

Properties: against colds, expectorant, anti-inflammatory, disinfectant (pseudomonas aeruginosa; promotes wound healing and scar formation.

Indications: chronic bronchitis and sinusitis, stomatitis, otitis, wounds, eczema.

Main components: D-fenchone, d-camphor, verbenone, alpha-pinene, camphene, cineole, linalool, Borneo Camphor.

Contraindications, side effects: avoid use for children and pregnant women, neurotoxic and abortive effect.

Lavandin Abrial:
Lavandula hybrida Briquet clone abrial (fl)—Labiatae

Properties: against infections, bacteria, fungi and viruses; general tonic; against colds, relieves coughs, sedative; promotes wound healing and scar formation.

Indications: ailments of respiratory tract, bronchitis, rhinopharyngitis, influenza; enterocolitis; rheumatism; asthenia; mycosis, wounds, skin ailments.
Main components: camphor, cineole, linaly acetate.
Contraindications, side effects: none known for normal dosage.

LAVANDIN GROSSO:
L. x Burnatii, Briquet clone grosso (fl)—Labiatae
Properties: against infection, bacteria, and fungi; general stimulant, especially for respiratory tract and digestive organs: analgesic: against rheumatism.
Indications: infection in throat-nose-ear area; atonic digestion; rheumatism, sciatica; insomnia.
Main components: linalyl acetate, linalool, camphor, cineole, terpineol-4.
Contraindications, side effects: none known for normal dosage.

LAVANDIN REYDOVAN:
L. x Buratii, Briquet clone reydovan (fl)—Labiatae
Properties: against microbes, bacteria, viruses, and fungi; tonic for body and nerves ; against colds, relieves coughs; sedative; promotes wound healing and scar formation.
Indications: complaints in throat-nose-ear area, bronchitis, influenza, rhinopharyngitis, coughing, sinusitis; digestive complaints, infectious enterocolitis; rheumatism; asthenia; mycosis, wounds, skin ailments.
Main components: linalyl acetate, linalool, camphor, 1-8-cineole, alpha- and beta-pinene, geraniol.
Contraindications, side effects: none known for normal dosage.

LAVANDIN SUPER:
Lavendula x Burnatii, Briquet clone super (fl)—Labiatae
Properties: against infection, bacteria, fungi, and viruses; general tonic; against colds, cough relief; analgesic, sedative; promotes wound healing and scar formation.
Indications: complaints in throat-nose-ear region, bronchitis, rhinopharyngitis, influenza, coughing; infectious enterocolitis; rheumatism, muscle rheumatism; asthenia; mycosis, wounds, skin ailments.
Main components: linalyl acetate, linalool, camphor, Borneo Camphor, 1-8-cineole.
Contraindications, side effects: none known for normal dosage.

LEEK:

Allium porrum L. (wp)—Liliaceae

Properties: strengthening, antiseptic for stomach-intestinal tract, purgative, diuretic; against rheumatism; nerve tonic.

Indications: digestive complaints, problems with food passage through intestines; complaints and stone problems in urinary tract; rheumatism, arthritis, gout; arteriosclerosis, corpulence; nervous exhaustion.

Main components: sulphur-nitrogen compounds.

Contraindications, side effects: irritant when applied externally.

LEMON:

Citrus limonum L (p)—Rutaceae

Properties: stimulating, strengthens heart and sympathetic nervous system; strengthens stomach, carminative, promotes urination, antiseptic and antibacterial; thins blood, alkalizing; against rheumatism; against sclerosis; vascular tonic; lowers blood pressure; promotes liver activity; against poisoning.

Indications: infectious diseases; asthenia; digestive complaints, hyperacidity (too much acid in stomach), aerophagy, liver insufficiency, kidney inflammation; inflammation of testicles; rheumatism, gout; vascular weakness, phlebitis; arteriosclerosis, high blood pressure; calcium deficiency, brittle nails; skin parasites, intestinal worms; malaria.

Main components: limonene, beta-pinen, gamma-terpinene.

Contraindications, side effects: skin irritation and photosensitizing when used externally.

LEMON BALM:

see *Melissa*

LEMON, CITRON:

Citrus medica L. (p)—Rutaceae

Properties: anti-infectious and anti-bacterial, antiseptic; promotes circulation, thins blood, dissolves stones, promotes digestion; nerve sedative; anti-inflammatory.

Indications: infections of respiratory tract, vascular weakness; liver and digestive weakness, kidney colic; nervous disorders, anxiety.

Main components: limonene, gamma-terpinene, alpha-pinene, geranial, neral, myrcene.

Contraindications, side effects: skin irritation and photosensitizing when used externally.

114

LEMONGRASS:
Cymbopogon citratus DC Stapf. Andropogon citratus D.C., Cymbopogon flexuosus Steud (wp)—Poaceae/Gramineae
Properties: stomach strengthening, stimulates appetite, promotes digestion, carminative; regulates vegetative nervous system, vascular expansion; against rickets; stimulant, anti-inflammatory, strong antiseptic, against parasites; febrifuge, diuretic.
Indications: atonic digestion, liver insufficiencies, cellulitis; infectious and feverish conditions; vegetative dystonia; arteritis, skin parasites.
Main components: citrals: neral, geranial; citronellal, methyl heptenone.
Contraindications, side effects: none known for normal dosage; dilute with plant when using externally to avoid strong skin irritation.

LEPTOSPERMUM:
see *Tea Tree, lemon*.

LIME, SWEET:
Citrus limetta Risso (p)—Rutaceae
Properties: stimulating and strengthening; stimulates appetite, carminative, diuretic; anti-spasmodic; antiseptic and anti-bacterial.
Indications: asthenia, insomnia; spasmic enterocolitis, flatulence, intestinal worms; skin parasites.
Main components: alpha-beta-pinene, furfural, d-limonene, linalyl acetate, linalool, dipentene, furcoumarin, auraptene, bergamotine, limettine.
Contraindications, side effects: photosensitizing and skin irritation when applied externally.

LINDEN:
Tilia sylvestris, Tilia europaea (fl + l)—Tiliaceae
The essential oil is acquired through synergistic co-distillation.
Properties: anti-spasmodic, sedative, diuretic; regulates circulation, expands blood vessels in head.
Linden Sapwood:
Tilia sylvestris (b)—Tiliaceae
The essential oil is acquired through synergistic co-distillation.
Properties: blood purifying, derivant for liver, gallbladder, and kidneys; diuretic, promotes urination; sedative, lowers blood pressure; against rheumatism; against cellulitis.

LOVAGE:

Levisticum officinalis Koch, Angelica levisticum Baillon, Ligusticum levisticum L. (r)—Apiaceae/Umbelliferae

Properties: stomach strengthening, promotes digestion, carminative, detoxifying for liver and gallbladder in particular, diuretic; blood purifying; nerve tonic, strengthens muscles (smooth vegetative musculature); anti-inflammatory and antifungal, against psoriasis; promotes menstruation, "anti-carcinogenic."

Indications: atony of digestive organs (stomach-liver-intestines), food poisoning, enterocolitis, consecutive symptoms of hepatitis, insufficient urination; chronic bronchitis; rheumatism, arthritis; mycosis, psoriasis, amenorrhea.

Main components: butylene acid, ligusteric acid, hexanol, d-alpha-terpineol, guaiacol, lupineol, bergaptene.

Contraindications, side effects: slightly irritating or possibility of photosensitizing when applied externally.

MACE:

Myristica fragrans Houtt. (seed hull that surrounds nutmeg)—Myristicaceae

Properties: strong stimulant and strengthening remedy; stimulates appetite; against asthma; against rheumatism; analgesic; against parasites.

Indications: atony of digestive organs, enterocolitis, diarrhea, flatulence, intestinal infection; acute and chronic rheumatism, joint pain, sprains, physical and mental asthenia, intestinal parasites.

Main components: beta-pinene, sabinene, myristicine, elemicine, camphene, p-cymene, d-linalool, Borneo Camphor, geraniol, safrol.

Contraindications, side effects: use internally only in weak dosages due to effect on nervous system; only for short periods of time.

MANDARIN:

Citrus reticulata Blanco, C. madurensis Lour. C. nobilis Lour (p)—Rutaceae

Properties: sedative, regulates the sympathetic nervous system, anti-spasmodic, analgesic, sleep remedy, against epilepsy; strengthens stomach, promotes digestion, promotes bile production; antibacterial and antifungal.

Indications: anxiety, neurasthenia, insomnia, shortness of breath, cardiovascular excitation; digestive complaints, aerophagy, hiccups, stomach pain; mycosis.

116

Main components: D-limonene, benzyl acetate, N-methyl anthranol acid, citrale.

Contraindications, side effects: photosensitizing and skin irritation when used externally.

MARJORAM, SWEET :

Origanum majorana L. (fl + l)—Labiatae

Properties: general strengthening, balancing of vegetative nervous system; vagotonic, stimulates the parasympathetic nervous system, subdues the sympathetic nervous systemj, regulates excessive functioning of thyroid gland; analgesic, sedative; lowers blood pressure through vasodilation, anaphrodisiac; anti-inflammatory and anti-bacterial; stomach strengthening, promotes digestion, carminative; promotes menstruation.

Indications: vegetative dystonia, high blood pressure, nervous disorders, asthenia, sexual sedative, runny nose, sinusitis, coughing, bronchitis, whooping cough, otitis; infections of digestive tract, nausea, and vomiting; rheumatism, arthrosis, neuralgia; amenorrhea.

Main components: d-alpha-terpineol, terpinene.

Contraindications, side effects: none known for normal dosage.

MARJORAM, WILD OR SPANISH MARJORAM

Thymus mastichina L. (fl + l)—Labiatae

Properties: against infection, bacteria, and viruses; against colds, expectorant, relieves coughs, reduces blockage of respiratory tract; stimulating and strengthening.

Indications: atony of respiratory and digestion, sinusitis, influenza, bronchitis, and viral bronchitis.

Main components: cineole, d-alpha-pinene, isovalerian acid, 1-linalool.

Contraindications, side effects: none known for normal dosage.

MASTIC TREE:

Pistacia lentiscus L. (l)—Anacardiaceae

Properties: reduces blood congestion in veins, lymph system, and prostate; diuretic; against asthma.

Indications: cardiovascular disturbances, hemorrhoids, varicose veins, little ruptured arteries, thrombo phlebitis; stomach ulcers, spasmic colitis, aerophagy; inflammation of prostate, sinusitis; asthma.

Main components: alpha-pinene, myrcene, terpenyl acetate.

Contraindications, side effects: none known for normal dosage.

MELALEUCA ALTERNIFOLIA:
see *Tea Tree*

MELALEUCA CAJEPUTII:
see *Cajeput*

MELALEUCA ERICIFOLIA:
(chemotype 1-8-cineole and linalool): Melaleuca ericifolia Sm. (1)—
Myrtaceae
Properties: against infection, bacteria, and viruses; relieves coughs, expectorant, soothing; anti-sclerotic.
Indications: infection of throat-nose-ear area, bronchitis, influenza, rhinopharyngitis; viral hepatitis and enterocolitis.
Main components: 1-8-cineole, linalool, terpinolene, terpinene, limonene, viridiflorene, alpha-terpineol.
Contraindications, side effects: none known for normal dosage.

MELALEUCA LEUCADENDRON:
see *Cajeput Leucadendron*.
Melaleuca Linarifolia:
Melaleuca linarifolia Smith (1)—Myrtaceae
Properties: anti-inflammatory, anti-bacterial and anti-viral; against colds, expectorant, relieves coughs; anti-sclerotic.
Indications: rhinopharyngitis, bronchitis, influenza; mammary tumor, viral liver and intestinal complaints.
Main components: 1-8-cineole, terpineol-1-4. terpinene.
Contraindications, side effects: none known for normal dosage.

MELALEUCA QUINQUENERVIA:
see under *Niaouli*

MELALEUCA UNCINATA:
Melaleuca uncinata R. Br. (1)—Myrtaceae
Properties: disinfectant, antibacterial, against parasites; anti-inflammatory; sedative, balances sympathetic and parasympathetic nervous system; expectorant, relieves coughs; wound healing.
Indications: bronchitis, pneumonia, sinusitis, asthma; inflamed and parasitic enterocolitis; bladder inflammation, urethra inflammation; wounds, skin ailments.

Main components: 1-8-cineole, alpha-pinene, alpha-terpineol, linalool, unceineol.
Contraindications, side effects: none known for normal dosage.

MELISSA OR LEMON BALM:
Melissa officinalis L. (fl + l)—Labiatae
Properties: anti-spasmodic, nerve calming, anti-depressant; stomach strengthening, stimulates appetite, promotes bile production; strengthens heart, stimulates body and mind (brain, heart, digestion, musculature, uterus); stops menstrual pain; anti-inflammatory, lowers blood pressure.
Indications: insomnia, nervousness, weak nerves, depressive anxiety; digestive complaints, upset stomach, migraines due to digestive disturbances, stomach cramps, liver-gallbladder insufficiency; nervous palpitations, epilepsy, dizziness attacks, ringing ears; cramping of respiratory tract and asthma.
Main components: neral, geranial, citronellal, geraniol, nerol, betacaryophyllene, alpha-copaene, alpha-humulene.
Contraindications, side effects: none known for normal dosage; by external use it can irritate sensitive skin.

MIMOSA:
Acacia decurrens (fl)—Mimosaceae
The essential oil is acquired through synergistic co-distillation.
Properties: blood purifier, derivant for liver and gallbladder, ailments of respiratory tract.

MINTS, VARIOUS TYPES
The mints possess a great capacity to crossbreed, producing diverse forms and sub-varieties. We attempt to present an overview of the main mint groups and a few of the unusual kinds:

- The water mints (M. aquatica L.)
- The green (spear) mints (M. viridis L.= M. spicata Huds), to which the Moroccan mint var. Nana belongs
- The field mints (M. arvensis L.)

Menta aquatica x viridis = peppermint (M. piperita L.)
There are three main forms of the peppermint:
- Mentha piperita vulgaris (sole) = the Mitcham mint with the main ingredient menthol

- Mentha piperita sylvestris (sole) = the Hungarian mint with the main ingredient menthone
- Mentha piperita officinalis (sole) = the white mint with the main components menthol and menthyl acetate

The unusual mint types are:
- European Pennyroyal (Mentha pulegium L.)
- Orange mint (Mentha citrata Ehrh.)
- Long-leafed mint (Mentha longifolia L./Huds)
- Apple mint (Mentha rotundifolia L./Huds), etc.

FIELD MINT:
Mentha arvensis L. (wp)—Labiatae

Properties: in weaker doses strengthening for digestion and heart; in stronger doses stimulating, then sedating; analgesic; promotes bile production and drainage of gallbladder; against circulatory disorders in head; antibacterial (staphylococci, meningococci), and anti-parasite.

Indications: nervous digestive disturbances, upset stomach, stomach ulcers, liver and kidney colics, constipation; migraines from digestive and circulatory disturbances; neuralgia, sciatica; rhinopharyngitis, sinusitis; worm diseases.

Main components: menthol, menthone, limonene, alpha-caryophyllene.

Contraindications, side effects: for babies and children under three years old, avoid internal and external application as well as inhalation.

NANA MINT OR MOROCCAN MINT:
Mentha viridis L. var. nana (l)—Labiatae

Properties: antibacterial, against viruses, fungi, and parasites; expectorant, against colds; against bruises, regenerative and healing for skin and mucous-membrane tissue.

Indications: bronchitis, influenza, sinusitis; sprains, hemorrhage, wounds; mycosis and parasitic skin ailments.

Main components: L-carvone, limonene, beta-caryophyllene, 1-8-cineole, myrcene.

Contraindications, side effects: avoid use by children and pregnant women because of ketone toxicity.

PEPPERMINT:
Mentha piperita L. (wp)—Labiatae

Properties: general strengthening and stimulating (brain, nerves, heart, kidneys, liver, pancreas, stomach, intestines); germicide for infections, bacteria, viruses, fungi, and worms; anti-inflammatory, promotes digestion, blood purifier; stops breast-milk production, regulates ovaries and promotes menstruation.

Indications: asthenia, vegetative dystonia, neuritis, headache, low blood pressure; aerophagy, stomach-intestine and liver-pancreas atony, colitis, kidney colic; bladder inflammation, prostate inflammation, vaginitis, leucorrhea; shingles, viral neuritis, yellow fever; sciatica, facial and dental neuralgia; nervous palpitations, dizziness, motion sickness, itchy irritation, skin parasites, intestinal worms.

Main components: menthol, menthone, menthyl acetate, 1-8-cineole, dimethyl sulfide.

Contraindications, side effects: avoid use by pregnant women and small children under three years old. Use externally, except for local application, because icy cold of the menthols.

PEPPERMINT *(Menthofurane chemotype):*
Mentha piperita L., M. sauvolens Ehrh. (wp)—Labiatae

Properties: against infection, bacteria, and fungi; against colds, expectorant, relieves coughing, anti inflammatory, analgesic; regulates heart; stimulates liver and urinary tract.

Indications: bronchitis, sinusitis, asthma, Vincent's angina; high blood pressure, cardiac irregularity, spasmophilia, Candida intestinal mycosis, liver insufficiency.

Main components: menthofurane, 1-8-cineole, alpha-beta-pinene, camphene, carvone.

Contraindications, side effects: none known.

PENNYROYAL, EUROPEAN:
Mentha pulegium L. (wp)—Labiatae

Properties: antiseptic, expectorant, relieves coughing; strengthens liver and spleen; stimulates appetite, carminative, sudorific; eases menstruation; "anti-carcinogenic."

Indications: liver-gallbladder complaints, bronchitis, chronic bronchitis, lung weakness; leucorrhea, painful or too strong menstruation; itching, skin parasites, intestinal worms.

Main components: pulegone, menthone, menthol.

Contraindications, side effects: avoid use by pregnant women and small children; don't use for longer period of time.

ORANGE MINT OR BERGAMOT MINT:
Mentha citrata Ehrh (wp)—Labiatae

Properties: anti-spasmodic, balancing for vegetative nervous system; anti-inflammatory; stimulates liver and pancreas; stimulant for ovaries as well as sexual stimulant; against parasites.

Indications: nervous exhaustion, tachycardia, digestive disorders and enterocolitis of nervous origin; inflamed bladder catarrh; liver-pancreas insufficiency, impotence; vermifuge, especially for maw-worm, amoebic dysentery.

Main components: linalool, linalyl acetate, terpineol, 1-8-cineole.

Contraindications, side effects: none known for normal dosage.

WOOD MINT:
Mentha sylvestris—M. longifolia L. (wp)—Labiatae

There is great variety of wood mints, and they all crossbreed easily. Depending on the area of growth, varieties with different chemical compositions can exist.

Properties: antiseptic, strengthening, antibacterial, antifungal; insufficiency of respiratory tract and digestive organs; stimulates the spleen, anti-spasmodic.

Indications: slow digestion, aerophagy; bronchitis; mycosis, bladder inflammation, Candida ailments, psoriasis.

Main components: piperitone oxide, linalyl acetate, alpha-murolene.

Contraindications, side effects: avoid use for children and pregnant women.

MUSTARD, BLACK:
Brassica nigra Koch., sinapsis alba, sinapsis juncea L., S. nigra Hooker (s)—Brassicaceae/Umbelliferae

Properties: derivant; reddens skin; analgesic, antifungal; antiseptic for intestinal and urinary tract; against tuberculosis; stimulates musculature and nerves.

Indications: general atony (brain, nerves, circulation, digestion, intestines, musculature), physical and mental asthenia, nervous depression; flatulence, spasmic and infectious enterocolitis, diarrhea, intestinal parasites; acute and chronic rheumatism, muscle cramps and muscle aches, sprains; paralysis; malaria; eases births; dental neuralgia, bad breath; skin parasites.

Main components: alpha-beta-pinene, sabinene, myrcene, alpha-gamma-terpinene, limonene, myristicine, camphene, p-cymene, d-linalool, Borneo Camphor, geraniol, elemicine, safrole.

Contraindications, side effects: for internal application use over a short time period or in weak dosage; can irritate the skin when used externally.

MUGWORT:
Artemisia aborescens L. (wp)—Asteraceae/Compositae
Properties: appetite stimulant, restorative, anti-asthmatic.
Caution: toxic in high doses!
Indications: slow digestion, asthenia; asthma and bronchitis; skin diseases.
Main components: azulene, chamazulene, Borneo Camphor, isovalerian-ester, perlargon-ester, limonene.
Contraindications, side effects: the dosage must be complied with exactly for internal use by children and pregnant women.

MUGWORT, COMMON:
Artemisia vulgaris L. (wp)—Asteraceae/Compositae
Properties: stimulates appetite, strengthening, anti-spasmodic, promotes bile flow, vermifuge; regulates female cycle, promotes menstruation.
Indications: menstruation: too strong, too weak or amenorrhea; loss of appetite, liver and gallbladder insufficiencies, worms.
Main components: alpha-thujone, camphor, cineole, delta-hydromatri-caria-ester.
Contraindications, side effects: the dosage must be complied with exactly for internal use by children and pregnant women.

MYRRH:
Commiphora myrrha Nees, C. abyssinica Engler (r)—Burseraceae
Properties: relieves coughs and sooths ailments of respiratory tract; strengthens, stimulates, anti-spasmodic; antiseptic, anti-inflammatory, against infection, viruses, and parasites; expansive, promotes wound healing and scar formation, regulates thyroid gland.
Indications: bronchitis, coughing, colds, asthma; diarrhea, dysentery, viral hepatitis; inflammation of urinary tract (bladder inflammation, inflammation of urethra); hyperfunction of thyroid gland; intestinal parasites (maw worm), skin ailments, skin ulcerations.
Main components: pinene, limonene, delta-beta-elemene, alpha-copaene, myrrhenic acid, cuminic, and cinnamaldehyde.
Contraindications, side effects: none known.

123

MYRTLE, COMMON (myrtenyl acetate-chemotype):
Myrtus communis L. (wp)—Myrtaceae
Properties: antiseptic for ailments of respiratory and urinary tract; sooths, anti-bacterial, prevents fermentation: astringent; hemostatic; anti-spasmodic; reduces blood congestion in veins and lymph vessels.
Indications: ailments of respiratory tract, colds, bronchitis; spasmic enterocolitis; bladder inflammation, urethra inflammation; hemorrhoids, varicose veins, enlarged lymph nodes.
Main components: myrtenyl acetate, 1-8-cineole, myrtenal, delta-cadinene.
Contraindications, side effects: none known for normal dosage.

MYRTLE, GREEN (cineole-chemotype):
Myrtus communis L. (wp)—Myrtaceae
Properties: against infections, against colds, expectorant, relieves coughs; stimulates liver, pancreas, and ovaries; reduces blood congestion in prostate anti-spasmodic, analgesic.
Indications: bronchitis, sinusitis, angina, muscovisidose; liver-gallbladder insufficiency; hypofunction of thyroid gland; amenorrhea; inflammation of prostate; insomnia; against facial wrinkles.
Main components: 1-8-cineole, alpha-pinene, azulene, humulene, dihydroazulene, linayl acetate, myrtenyl acetate.
Contraindications, side effects: none known for normal dosage.

NEROLI (BITTER ORANGE BLOSSOM):
Citrus bigaradia Risso, C. aurantium L. ssp amara (fl)—Rutaceae
The essential oil of the orange blossom comes either from the sweet orange (var. aurantium) or from the bitter orange (var. bigaradia). Its contents and therefore its properties are related. There are however certain differences between the two sorts, dependent on the origin.
Properties: analgesic, anti-spasmodic, stimulates appetite; heart tonic, mild sedative and soporific; blood purifier, detoxifying; beneficial effect on skin; against infection, bacteria, and parasites; tonic for digestion, veins, brain, and nerves; lowers blood pressure, "anti-carcinogenic."
Indications: nervous depression, exhaustion, heart pounding, high blood pressure, insomnia; liver-pancreas insufficiency; plethora, diarrhea, enterocolitis through bacteria and parasites (hook worm and Lamblia); hemorrhoids, varicose veins, phlebitis; skin care.
Main components: jasmone, linalyl acetate, farnesol, linalool, geranieol, nerolidol, alpha-terpineo, nerol, dipentene.
Contraindications, side effects: none known for normal dosage.

NIAOULI (cineole-chemotype):
Melaleuca quinquenervia(Cav.) cineolifera (l)—Myrtaceae
Properties: against infection, bacteria, viruses, and fungi; sooths, against colds, expectorant, relieves coughs, anti-inflammatory, febrifuge, anti-allergic; lowers blood pressure; general stimulant, especially for the tissue, liver, bladder, the reticulo-endothelial terrain, estrogen production, and hypophysic-testicles; reduces blood congestion in veins, dissolves stones; against tumors; protects skin during radiation therapy, promotes wound healing and scar formation.

Indications: infection in throat-nose-ear area, in stomach-intestinal tract, and in uro-genital system; bronchitis and chronic colds, tuberculosis, rhinopharyngitis, sinusitis, tonsil inflammation; blepharitis; enteritis and viral hepatitis, cholera, diarrhea, stomach and duodenal ulcers, gallstones; arteritis, coronary inflammation, endocarditis, atherosclerosis, hemorrhoids, urethra-prostate inflammations, vaginitis, dysplasia of cervix, genital herpes; condyloma, support for breast and rectal cancer, rheumatic polyarthritis; psoriasis, boils, skin inflammation, leprosy, mycosis, wounds, bites, radiation therapy, and burns from electro-coagulation (external).

Main components: 1-8-cineole, viridiflorol, alpha-terpineol, alpha-beta-pinene, limonene, globulol, neridol.

Contraindications, side effects: none known for normal dosage. Use weak dosages internally for children and pregnant women.

NIAOULI (transnerolidol-chemotype):
Melaleuca quinquenervia (Cac.) transnerolidolifera (l)—Myrtaceae
Properties: antibacterial, against virus and parasites; sedative; anti-inflammatory for respiratory tract and uro-genital system; stimulates the hypophysic-testicles and hypophysic suprarenal cortex (according to P. Franchomme, D. Pénoel).

Indications: bronchitis, sinusitis; viral hepatitis, parasitic enterocolitis, digestive complaints; malaria; bladder and urethra inflammations; high blood pressure; arthrosis, rheumatic polyarthritis; asthenia, exhaustion; shingles, eczema.

Main components: transnerolidol, linalool, alpha-terpineol, beta-caryophyllene, alpha-humulene, delta-cadinene.

Contraindications, side effects: careful doses for internal use by women.

In Australia there is a large variety of Melaleucas. As for the types of Niaouli, the various chemotypes of Melaleuca quinquenervia will be studied more carefully in a later edition.

NIAOULI (linalool chemotype):
Melaleuca quinquenervia (Cav.) linalolifera (l)—Myrtaceae
Main components: linalool (~59%), transnerolidol (20%).
Niaouli (viridiflorol chemotype):
Melaleuca quinquenervia (Cav.) viridiflorulifera (l)—Myrtaceae
Main components: 1-8-cineole (39%), viridiflorol (24%), transnerolidol, limonene, alpha-terpineol.

NUTMEG:
Myristica fragrans Houtt. (nut)—Myristicaceae
Properties: general remedy for energy-strengthening and stimulating, especially for brain and circulation; against asthenia; stomach strengthening, stimulates appetite, promotes digestion, speeds up passage of food, promotes menstruation; against infections, antiseptic, analgesic, anesthetic; muscle tonic, softening, lowers blood pressure; sedative, antidepressant, against rheumatism; against parasites.
Indications: general atony (brain, nerves, circulation, digestion, intestines, musculature), physical and mental asthenia, nervous depression; flatulence, spasmic and infectious enterocolitis, diarrhea, intestinal parasites; acute and chronic rheumatism, muscle cramps, sprains; paralysis; eases birth; dental neuralgia, bad breath, skin parasites.
Main components: alpha-beta-pinene, sabinene, myrcene, alpha-gamma-terpinene, limonene, myristicine, camphene, p-cymene, d-linalool, Borneo Camphor, geraniol, elemicine, safrol.
Contraindications, side effects: use internally for short periods or in weak dosage, can cause skin irritation when used externally.

ONION:
Allium cepa L. (bulb)—Liliaceae
Properties: antiseptic, against infection, slows bacterial multiplication; lowers blood sugar; strongly diuretic, helps eliminate urine and chloride; general stimulant for nervous system; promotes bile production and drainage of gallbladder; relieves coughs; reduces blood congestion in pelvic region; heart strengthening; regulates glandular function; against sclerosis; against scrofulsis; promotes hair growth; aphrodisiac.
Indications: infection of respiratory tract; cardiac insufficiency, pericarditis; arteriosclerosis; physical and mental asthenia; infectious colitis; diabetes; corpulence, plethora, prostate inflammation, insufficient urination, edema; rheumatism, arthritis, gout; intestinal parasites; abscess, boils, panaritium (pus-infected fingers).

Main components: disulfide, allyl sulfide, dipropyl-trisulfide.
Contraindications, side effects: skin irritation when applied externally.

OPOPONAX:
Opoponax chironiu, (L.) Koch, Commiphora erythraea var. glabrescens Engler (r)—Burseraceae/Apiaceae
Properties: derivant, detoxifying, stimulates liver and kidneys.
Indications: plethora, toxemia, liver and kidney atony, skin rash, skin ailments.
Main components: bisabolene, phthalide, sesquiterpenone.
Contraindications, side effects: none known.

ORANGE, BITTER:
Citrus aurantium L. var. amara Link. (p)—Rutaceae
Properties: sedative; anti-spasmodic; stimulates digestion; anti-coagulant, thinning.
Indications: anxiety, nervousness, asthenia, dizziness; digestive complaints, flatulence, stomach cramps, plethora, toxemia; circulatory weakness and venous stasis.
Main components: limonene, terpinolene, d-alpha-terpineol, d-l-linalool, geraniol, citronellol, terpinolene, nerolidol, farnesol.
Contraindications, side effects: photosensitizing when used externally.

ORANGE, BLOOD:
Citrus sinensis L. (p)—Rutaceae
Properties and indications are very similar to Sweet Orange.

ORANGE BLOSSOM:
see *Neroli*.

ORANGE, SWEET:
Citrus sinensis L. (p)—Rutaceae
Properties: sedative, analgesic, anti-spasmodic; promotes digestion, purgative, blood purifying, diuretic, stimulates heart and circulation; antiseptic.
Indications: anxiety, neurasthenia, insomnia; digestive complaints, constipation; circulatory weakness; air disinfectant.
Main components: D-limonene, terpinolene, alpha-terpinene, citrale, furocoumarin, carvone, linalool, beta-carotene.
Contraindications, side effects: photosensitizing when applied externally.

127

ORIGANUM, GREEN:
Origanum heracleot. L. (wp + fl)—Lamiaceae/Labiatae
Properties and indications similar to Moroccan Origanum.
Main components: carvacrol, thymol, p-cymene.

ORIGANUM, MOROCCAN:
Origanum compactum Bentham (wp + fl)—Lamiaceae/Labiatae
Properties: strong disinfectant with broad spectrum, antibacterial, antiviral, antifungal; general physical and mental tonic; anti-inflammatory; stimulates immune system.
Indications: infection processes of respiratory tract, entire digestive tract, and uro-genital system; upset stomach, diarrhea, amoebic dysentery, malaria; kidney inflammation; neuritis; low blood pressure; physical and nervous asthenia; skin parasites.
Main components: carvacrol, thymol, alpha-beta-pinene, myrcene, p-cymene, geraniol.
Contraindications, side effects: irritates the liver when used internally; should be applied either in strong dosage for short use or in weaker dosage for longer use; caustic for the skin when used externally.

ORIGANUM, SPANISH (CANDLEWOOD):
Corydothymus capitatus L. (fl)—Lamiaceae/Labiatae
Properties: strong disinfectant with broad spectrum, antibacterial, antiviral, antifungal; general physical and mental tonic.
Indications: infection processes of respiratory tract, the entire digestive tract, and uro-genital system; asthenia, low blood pressure; abscess, skin parasites.
Main components: carvacrol, thymol, beta-caryophyllene, Borneo Camphor, dipentene, bornyl acetate.
Contraindications, side effects: irritates the liver when used internally; should be applied either in strong dosage for short use or in weaker dosage for longer use; caustic for the skin when used externallyj.

PALMAROSA:
Cymbopogon martinii Stapf. (wp)—Gramineae
Properties: important anti-bacterial remedy, antifungal and antiviral; strengthens digestion, uterus, nerves, and heart; febrifuge; stimulates cells for skin and hair care (hydrates, freshens); vermifuge.
Indications: rhinopharyngitis, sinusitis, otitis, bronchitis; dyspepsia, bacterial and viral intestinal inflammation; urethra inflammation, bladder inflammation, vaginitis; eases birth; acne, dry and wet eczema.

Main components: geraniol, linalool, geranyl formiate, geranyl acetate.
Contraindications, side effects: none known for normal dosage.

PARSLEY:
Petroselinum sativum Hoffm. (s)—Apiaceae/Umbelliferae
Properties: general strengthening for brain, uterus, and musculature; effect similar to estrogen, regulates menstruation; antiseptic for respiratory tract and uro-genital system.
Indications: asthenia; physical, muscular, and mental exhaustion; infections and insufficiency of uro-genital system, urethra inflammation, leucorrhea, amenorrhea; infrequent menstruation or amenorrhea; asthma.
Main components: apiol, myristicine, alpha-pinene, apiine, allyl-1-tetramethoxyl benzol.
Contraindications, side effects: children and pregnant women should not use it.

PARSLEY, SMOOTH:
Petroselinum sativum Hoffm., apium petrolinum L. (wp)—Apiaceae/Umbelliferae
Properties: general tonic, stomach strengthening; derivant, diuretic, blood purifying; anti-spasmodic.
Indications: asthenia, atony of digestive organs and kidneys; rheumatism, gout; menstrual complaints; neurasthenia.
Main components: alpha-beta-pinene, myristicine, beta-phellandrene, terpinolene, isopropenyl-4-benzol, p-menthatriene.
Contraindications, side effects: children and pregnant women should not use it.

PATCHOULI:
Pogostemon patchouli Pell., P. suavis Ten., P. cablin Benth. (wp)—Labiatae
Properties: antiseptic, anti-inflammatory, reduces blood congestion; against infection, antibacterial, antifungal; insect repellant; febrifuge; wound healing, regenerates tissue, strengthening, especially for the veins; against women's diseases.
Indications: infectious enterocolitis, bladder inflammation, vaginitis, urethra inflammation; hemorrhoids, varicose veins; eczema, acne, inflamed skin ailments, scabs, chapping, skin parasites.
Main components: patchoulol, alpha-beta-bulnesene, patchoulene, seychellene, pogostol, patchouli pyridine, azulene.
Contraindications, side effects: none known for normal dosage.

PEMOU:
Fokienia Hodginsii Henry and Thomas, Cupressus hodginsii Dunn. F. kaway B. Hayata (w)—Cupressaceae
Properties: strengthening, neurotonic, stimulates hypophsic-testicles and suprarenal cortex.
Indications: exhaustion, asthenia, impotence (in men).
Main components: trans-nerolidol, focienol, elemol.
Contraindications, side effects: should not be used by women.

PEPPER, BLACK:
Piper nigrum L. (fruit)—Piperaceae
Properties: stimulates digestive and respiratory tract; expectorant, relieves coughs; against asthenia; carminative; febrifuge, analgesic, antiseptic for urinary tract; aphrodisiac.
Indications: weak digestion, insufficiency of liver, pancreas, and intestines; angina; larynx inflammation; chronic bronchitis; bladder inflammation; dental neuralgia; rheumatic pain; cerebral and sexual asthenia.
Main components: beta-caryophyllene, alpha-humulene, alpha-guajene, selinene, cubebene, elemene, bisabolene, alpha-beta-pinene, phellandrene, piperonal, Borneo Camphor, chavicol.
Contraindications, side effects: none known.

PERU BALSAM:
Myroxylon balsamum var. pereirae Miller (r)—Coniferae
Properties: sooths and antiseptic for ailments of respiratory tract and bronchial complaints; antiseptic for urinary tract, diuretic; antibacterial against parasites; promotes wound healing and scar formation; for skin ailments; against rheumatism; analgesic.
Indications: mainly for external use—for bronchitis, influenza, coughing, tuberculosis; bladder inflammation, urethra inflammation, vaginitis; itching, irritation, skin ailments, skin parasites; rheumatic pain.
Main components: cinnamic and benzoic acid, nerolidol, benzyl benzoate, cinnamic acid benzyl-ester.
Contraindications, side effects: can irritate when used over longer period of time.

PETITGRAIN (BITTER ORANGE):
Citrus aurantium L. ssp. amara, ssp. aurantium (l)—Rutaceae
Properties: sedative to nervous system beneath the diaphragm; anti-spasmodic; anti-inflammatory; anti-bacterial.

130

Indications: vegetative dystonia; infections of respiratory tract; acne with pus, boils; chronic hepatitis.
Main components: linalyl acetate, 1-linalool, alpha-terpineol, nerol, geraniol, furfal, beta-ocimene, dipentene.
Contraindications, side effects: none known for normal dosage.

PETITGRAIN (COMBAVA):
Combava hystrix DC (fl)—Rutaceae
Properties: sedative, anti-inflammatory; analgesic; against rheumatism.
Indications: nervousness, anxiety, insomnia; rheumatism, arthritis.
Main components: citronellal, linalool, citronellol.
Contraindications, side effects: none known.

PETITGRAIN (LEMON TREE):
Citrus limonum L. (l)—Rutaceae
Properties: sedates nervous system beneath the diaphragm; promotes digestion; antiseptic.
Indications: vegetative dystonia, atony of digestion and pancreas.
Main components: pinene, limonene, linalool, geraniol.
Contraindications, side effects: none known for normal dosage.

PETITGRAIN (MANDARIN):
Citrus reticulata Blanco (l)—Rutaceae
Properties: general sedative, anti-spasmodic, analgesic.
Indications: anxiety, stress, atonic digestion of nervous origin, insomnia.
Main components: pinene, limonene, dipentene, p-cymene, geraniol, N-methyl anthranylate.
Contraindications, side effects: none known for normal dosage.

PINE, AUSTRIAN BLACK:
Pinus nigra Arnold austiaca (n)—Abietaceae/Pinaceae
Properties: germicide for the air and respiratory tract, expectorant; stimulating; against rheumatism.
Indications: infection of respiratory tract, bronchitis, sinusitis; asthenia, exhaustion; rheumatism, skin ailments; freshens and disinfects the air.
Main components: 1-alpha-pinene, d-limonene, 1-cadinene, beta-pinene.
Contraindications, side effects: none known for normal dosage; can be irritating to skin and mucous membranes if not diluted.

PINE, BEACH:

Pinus pinaster Soland. (n)—Abietaceae/Pinaceae

Properties: antiseptic, protects the mucous membranes of bronchial tract and uro-genital system; strengthening, circulatory tonic; germicide for the air.

Indications: bronchitis, sinusitis; chronic bladder inflammation; circulatory disturbances; disinfects room air.

Main components: alpha- and beta-pinene, delta 3-carene, terpineolene, beta-caryophyllene, Borneo Camphor.

Contraindications, side effects: None known for normal dosage, but take in weak doses for internal applications.

PINE, BEACH:

Pinus pinaster Soland. (b)—Abietaceae/Pinaceae

Properties: germicide for respiratory tract and uro-genital system; anti-inflammatory for respiratory tract, kidneys, and joints.

Indications: sinusitis, chronic bronchitis; chronic bladder inflammation; rheumatism.

Main components: alpha- and beta-pinene.

Contraindications, side effects: None known for normal dosage.

PINE, CORSICAN BLACK:

Pinus nigra Lk. ssp laricio Poiret (n)—Abietaceae

Properties: antiseptic for respiratory tract and chest cavity, for coughs; strengthening and stimulating; reduces blood congestion in lymph vessels and prostate.

Indications: bronchitis, sinusitis; exhaustion, asthenia, swelling of prostate.

Main components: alpha-beta-pinene, limonene, Borneo Camphor and bornyl acetate, larichiol.

Contraindications, side effects: none known for normal dosage.

PINE, DWARF OR MOUNTAIN:

Pinus mughus Scop. var. P. pumilio Turra.Haencke, P. uncinata Mirb. (n)—Abietaceae/Pinaceae

Properties: against infection of respiratory tract; antibacterial, germicide for the air; anti-inflammatory; against arthrosis; dissolves stones; general strengthening.

Indications: bronchitis, sinusitis, pleurisy, tuberculosis; gallbladder inflammation, gallstones; rheumatism, arthrosis; asthenia; skin diseases.

Main components: alpha-beta-pinene, 1-phellandrene, 1-limonene, silvestrene, bornyl acetate, Borneo Camphor. pumiliol, cadinene, anise aldehyde.

Contraindications, side effects: none known for normal dosage.

PINE, GENERAL OR SCOTS:

Pinus sylvestris L. (n)—Abietaceae/Pinaceae

Properties: tonic, general physical, nerve stimulant and sexual stimulant; raises blood pressure; against infection, anti-bacterial, anti-fungal, anti-inflammatory; against diabetes; effect similar to cortisone; pituitary gland-suprarenal connection (according to P. Franchomme-D. Penéol), reduces blood congestion in lymph glands and uro-genital system; against arthritis.

Indications: exhaustion, asthenia, convalescence; bronchitis, chronic bronchitis, sinusitis, asthma; inflammatory processes; rheumatism, rheumatic polyarthritis; multiple sclerosis; uterine congestion, kidney inflammation.

Main components: alpha-beta-pinene, limonene, bornyl acetate, Borneo Camphor.

Contraindications, side effects: none known for normal dosage.

PINE, SEA:

Pinus halepensis Mill. (n)—Abietaceae/Pinaceae

Properties: germicide for the air; sedative, analgesic; soothing, against infection of respiratory tract; against rheumatism; general stimulant.

Indications: bronchitis, colds, sinusitis, asthma; rheumatism; atony of respiratory tract and circulatory system; freshens and disinfects room air.

Main components: D-alpha-pinene, bornyl acetate, Borneo Camphor, caryophyllene, dipentene, phenyl ethylalochol.

Contraindications, side effects: none known for normal dosage; can cause irritation of skin or mucous membranes when not diluted.

PINE, SIBERIAN:

Abies sibirica Ledeb, Picea obovata Ledeb, Abies pichte Fisch/Forb (n)—Abietaceae

Properties: sedative, anti-spasmodic, anti-inflammatory, against infection of respiratory tract.

Indications: nervous disorders, agitation; inflammatory processes; muscle rheumatism; suppuration of tooth root.

Main components: bornyl acetate, terpineol, alpha-beta pinene, 1-camphene, alpha-phellandrene, bisabolene, isoborneol.
Contraindications, side effects: none known for normal dosage.

RAVENSARA:
Ravensara aromatica JF. Cimel/Sonnerat (l)—Lauraceae
Properties: against infection, antibacterial, and antiviral; antitoxic; stimulates immune system; general strengthening and stimulating, while at the same time sedative and analgesic.
Indications: influenza, rhinopharyngitis, sinusitis, bronchitis, whooping cough; viral hepatitis, viral enteritis, cholera, herpes, shingles, chicken pox; infectious mononucleosis (lymphoid cell angina), blood poisoning, plague; asthenia, neuromuscular atony and complaints, irritability, insomnia.
Main components: alpha-beta-pinene, 1-8-cineole, beta-caryophyllene, alpha-terpineol, terpenyl acetate, chavicol.
Contraindications, side effects: none known for normal dosage.

RAVENSARA, ANISE:
Ravensara anisata Danguy (b)—Lauraceae
Properties: sedative, anti-spasmodic, analgesic, moderate regulating effect; promotes menstruation, builds breast-milk through estrogen similarity; stimulant and strengthening for respiratory tract and digestion, carminative, promotes production of bile and drainage of gallbladder; strengthens heart.
Indications: weak nerves, spasmophilia, paralysis; painful, weak, and irregular menstruation; during breast-feeding; complaints of menopause; nervous dyspepsia, asthma, lung congestion; digestive complaints, stomach pain, spasmic colitis, flatulence; nervous palpitations, cardiovascular arythmia.
Main components: anethol, methyl-ether-chavicol, sesquiterpene.
Contraindications, side effects: avoid use for children and pregnant women.

ROSE, DAMASCUS:
Rosa damascaena Miller, Rosa centifolia L. (fl)—Rosaceae
Properties: toning for heart, stomach, liver, and uterus; strengthening, astringent, expectorant; slight laxative; promotes wound healing and scar formation; hemostatic, antiseptic, and anti-inflammatory; antiviral and antibacterial; sedative, strengthens nerves; aphrodisiac.
Indications: chronic bronchitis and angina, tuberculosis, asthma; nervousness; sexual asthenia, frigidity, impotence; exhaustion, atony; skin ailments,

wounds, inflammatory processes, atonic ulcers; sprains, strains; little ruptured arteries, facial wrinkles, skin care; aphtha, gum inflammation.

Main components: phenylethyl alcohol, geraniol, citronellal, nerol, rhodinol.

Contraindications, side effects: none known for normal dosage.

ROSEMARY, BUSH *(verbenone chemotype):*
Rosmarinus officinalis L. (wp + fl)—Lamiaceae/Labiatae

Properties: against infection, antibacterial and antiviral; against colds, expectorant; relieves coughs; anti-spasmodic; disinfectant and stimulating effect on liver and gallbladder; balancing for nerves, endocrine system, and hypophysic ovaries or testicles.

Indications: bronchitis, sinusitis; viral hepatitis and hepatitis caused by colibacteria; cholera; vaginitis, leucorrhea; exhaustion, nervous depression; relaxing for solar plexus, pelvis, and sacrum (arhythmia, tachycardia, digestive and sexual problems).

Main components: verbenone, 1-8-cineole, alpha-pinene, Borneo Camphor, camphene, myrcene, limonene, alpha-terpinene.

Contraindications, side effects: avoid use by small children, pregnant women, and people with hypersensitive livers.

ROSEMARY, CINEOLE AND PROVENCE PYRAMID ROSEMARY *(cineole chemotype):*
Rosmarinus officinalis L. cineoliferum—R. pyramidalis (wp + fl)—Lamiacae/Labiatae

Properties: against infection, antibacterial, antifungal; against colds, expectorant, relieves coughs; general mild stimulant, especially for respiratory tract, circulation, liver and digestive system.

Indications: otitis, sinusitis, bronchitis, colds, pneumonia; rheumatic neuralgia, neurasthenia; digestive complaints, nausea, enterocolitis caused by fermentation processes; bladder inflammation; Candida fungal diseases, leucorrhea, spermatorrhea; exhaustion.

Main components: 1-8-cineole, alpha-beta-pinene, camphene, beta-caryophyllene, Borneo Camphor, bornyl acetate, camphor.

Contraindications, side effects: none known for normal dosage.

ROSEMARY, SPANISH CAMPHOR *(camphor chemotype):*
Rosmarinus off. L. camphoriferum (wp + fl)—Lamiaceae/Labiatae

Properties: general tonic (brain, nerves, muscles, liver, gallbladder, heart, respiratory tract); stimulates bile production and drainage of gallbladder;

135

expectorant; diuretic; reduces blood congestion in veins; promotes menstruation; for hyperthermia.

Indications: physical, mental, and muscular asthenia; muscle tension and cramping, muscle rheumatism, rheumatic neuralgia, agitated progressive paralysis; cardiac insufficiency, nervous palpitations; venous stasis, varicose veins, lower blood pressure (in very weak doses. brings blood pressure into equilibrium); digestive complaints, nausea, chronic gallbladder inflammation, liver cirrhosis; hyperchloesteremia; amenorrhea, leucorrhea, spermatorrhea; sensitivity to cold.

Main components: camphor, 1-8-cineole, alpha-pinene, camphene, Borneo Camphor, beta-caryophyllene.

Contraindications, side effects: none known for normal dosage.

ROSEWOOD:

Aniba rosaeodora Ducke var. amazonica, Aniba parviflora Mez. (w)—Lauraceae

Properties: antiseptic and disinfectant, antibacterial, antiviral, antifungal, and against parasites; sexually strengthening; beneficial effect on the skin, fine perfume.

Indications: infections in throat-nose-ear area and bronchial-lung area; influenza; vaginitis through Candida; depression, asthenia, overexertion; frigidity, impotence; skin problems, skin ailments, mycosis, acne, facial wrinkles, etc.

Main components: linalool, terpineol, geraniol, dipentene, eucalyptol, methyl heptenol, nerol.

Contraindications, side effects: none known for normal dosage.

RUE:

Ruta graveolens L. (wp)—Rutaceae

Properties: promotes menstruation (abortive); sudorific; anti-spasmodic; stimulates vascular circulation (rutine content); against rheumatism; vermifuge.

Indications: vascular circulatory problems; rheumatism; skin parasites, ailments due to worms.

Main components: L-4-pinene, 1-limonene, cineole, methyl-nonylephytl-ketone, salicylic acid.

Contraindications, side effects: avoid internal use without medical follow-up (very poisonous effect on nerves and strongly abortive).

136

SAGE, CLARY:

Salvia sclarea L. (wp)—Lamiaceae/Labiatae

Properties: effects hormonal-genital system (scareol = similar to estrogen), promotes menstruation, aphrodisiac; stimulates circulation, strengthens veins; anti-spasmodic, sedative, against epilepsy; stimulates medulla oblongata and cerebellum; fights deterioration of cells; lowers cholesterol; antifungal; reduces sweat production; stimulates hair growth.

Indications: amenorrhea, pre-menopause, genital complaints associated with hormonal weakness; circulatory disturbances; varicose veins, hemorrhoids, vein expansion; agitated and nervous exhaustion; high cholesterol level; mycosis; hair loss.

Main components: linayl acetate, linalool, furfurol, sclareol, beta caryo phyllene, germacrene.

Contraindications, side effects: mastitis; carcinous. Do not take together with medications containing iron.

SAGE, COMMON:

Salvia officinalis L. (wp + fl)—Lamiaceae/Labiatae

Properties: general stimulant; against infection, antibacterial, antiviral, antifungal; febrifuge; against colds, expectorant, relieves coughs; splits fat (against cellulitis); stimulates circulation; limits sweat production; stomach strengthening, stimulates bile production and drainage of gallbladder; promotes menstruation; promotes wound healing and scar formation.

Indications: exhaustion, convalescence, psychoasthenia; meningitis and viral neuritis; influenza, bronchitis, angina, sinusitis; aphtha ailments, herpes; digestive complaints, viral enteritis, gallbladder insufficiency; rheumatic polyarthritis; insufficient urination; cellulitis, circulatory disturbances; amenorrhea, pre-menopause, leucorrhea, spermatorrhea,; condyloma, wounds, skin ailments, hair loss.

Main components: alpha-beta-thujon, camphor, 1-8-cineole, lanalol, a-terpineol, humulene, Borneo Camphor, beta-caryophyllene, alpha-beta-pinene, camphene.

Contraindications, side effects: should not be used by children and pregnant women due to ketone toxicity.

Remarks:
1. The content of alpha-thujone, which consists of 25—30% during the harvest in spring, can double in the autumn to 50—60%.
2. Traditionally, garden sage has been considered to have a beneficial effect on conception. This effect is certainly associated with its stimu-

lating properties and their similarities to hormones. However, it should not be recommended for this purpose because of its high content of thujone, which has abortive properties. It is also true that small-leafed sage of the chemotype 1-8-cineole, which has ten times less thujone, replaces classic garden sage in a beneficial way for this type of use. It is also recommended for every type of internal application for children or pregnant women, who should be monitored by an aromatherapist.

SAGE, GREEK:

Salvia fructicosa Mill. (wp + fl)—Lamiaceae/Labiatae
Properties: against colds, relieves coughs, expectorant; against infections, antiviral; stimulating.
Indications: bronchial colds and chronic bronchitis, rhinopharyngitis, sinusitis; chronic cold infections (leucorrhea); vaginitis; states of exhaustion.
Main components: 1-8-cineole, alpha-and beta-pinene, myrcene, camphene, beta-caryophyllene, alpha-humulene, Borneo Camphor, fenchone, camphor.
Contraindications, side effects: avoid use by small children and pregnant women.

SAGE, LAVENDER-LEAFED GARDEN:

Salvia lavandulifolia Vahl. (wp + fl)—Lamiaceae/Labiatae
Properties: general stimulant and strengthening; antiseptic, against infection; against colds, relieves coughs; analgesic.
Indications: asthenia, psychoasthenia; bronchitis, influenza, sinusitis; colds, neuralgia.
Main components: 1-8-cineole, linalool, delta-terpineol, Borneo Camphor, alpha-beta-pinene, camphene, myrcene, many sesquiterpenes, alpha-cubebene, alpha-copaene, beta-caryophellene, alpha-humulene, etc.
Contraindications, side effects: none known for normal dosage.

SAGE, SMALL-LEAFED (CHEMOTYPE 1-8-CINEOLE):

Salvia officinalis Drome (wp + fl)—Lamiaceae/Labiatae
Properties: general strengthening; stimulating for the body and mind; against infection, antibacterial; against colds, expectorant, relieves coughs; general derivant, analgesic, sedative; promotes wound healing.
Indications: general exhaustion, post-traumatic or post-operative exhaustion; convalescence; chronic bronchitis, angina, influenza, rhinopharyn-

gitis, sinusitis; toxicity of humoral terrain; nervousness, insomnia; skin ailments, wounds.

Main components: 1-8-cineole, camphor, alpha-beta-pinene, camphene, humulene, Borneo Camphor, alpha-thujone.

Contraindications, side effects: should be avoided by pregnant women and infants.

SANDALWOOD, WHITE:
Santalum album L. (r)—Santalaceae

Properties: antiseptic for uro-genital system; against gonorrhea; diuretic; stimulating and strengthening; aphrodisiac; reduces blood congestion in venous stasis; astringent; against diarrhea; skin care, against acne; as perfume.

Indications: infection of uro-genital system (gonorrhea, bladder inflammation, diseases caused by colibacteria, leucorrhea); sexual atony; circulatory disturbances; venous stasis (minor pelvis); varicose veins, hemorrhoids; cardiac insufficiency; chronic bronchitis; diarrhea; sciatica, lumbago; beneficial for the skin.

Main components: alpha-beta-santalol, santalene, pinene, phellandrene.

Contraindications, side effects: none known for normal dosage.

SANTOLINA:
Santolina chamaecyparissus L. (wp)—Asteraceae/Compositae

Properties: vermifuge (ascaridene, oxyurene); against infections, antifungal; expectorant, against colds; stimulating; anti-inflammatory; promotes menstruation.

Indications: vermifuge (askaridene, etc.), skin parasites.

Main components: 1-iso-artemisi acetone, santolinenone, alpha-beta-pinene.

Contraindications, side effects: avoid all uses for children and pregnant women (neurotoxic and abortive effect).

SASSAFRAS:
Sassafras off. S. albidum (Nutt.) Nees (North America)—Cinnamomum micranth. Hayater (China)—Ocotea pretiosa Nees (Brazilian) (b + w + r)—Lauraceae

Properties: against infection, antibacterial; antiseptic for uro-genital system; strengthening, stimulating, diuretic, carminative; analgesic; against rheumatism; reduces blood pressure; remedy against tobacco (according to Shelby).

Indications: complaints of respiratory tract and uro-genital system; calculosis and kidney pain, bladder inflammation, leucorrhea; rheumatic neuralgia, arthritis, gout, sciatica, lumbago, muscle pain, lumbar pain; asthenia; arterial high blood pressure, skin ailments caused by parasites (mites, lice).

Main components: safrol, cadinene, alpha-pinene, phellandrene, d-camphor, eugenol, cetiol.

Contraindications, side effects: should be avoided by children and pregnant women (compare with note on safrol in the chart "Biochemical Elements of Essential Oils").

SAVIN:
see *Juniper*

SAVORY, GARDEN:
Satureja hortensis L. (wp + fl)—Labiatae

Properties: very effective against infection, antibacterial, antiviral, antifungal, against parasites; physical and mental strengthening; strengthening and stimulation of digestive and intestinal tracts; raises blood pressure; against rheumatism.

Indications: infectious and viral diseases in overall organism; physical, nervous, and sexual asthenia; low blood pressure; rheumatism; mycosis.

Main components: carvacrol, alpha-beta-terpenes, p-zymene, thymol, b-caryophyllene, cineole.

Contraindications, side effects: caution recommended when using externally (very localized); caustic effect on skin and mucous membranes.

SAVORY, MOUNTAIN:
Satureja montana L. (wp + fl)—Labiatae

Properties: very effective against infection, antibacterial, antiviral, antifungal, against parasites; stimulates immune resistance, physical and mental strengthening and stimulation (nervous system, circulation, digestion, and intestinal tract); raises blood pressure; against rheumatism; anti-inflammatory, analgesic.

Indications: bronchitis, tuberculosis, influenza, sinusitis; digestive problems, enteritis, and enterocolitis; diarrhea, amoebic dysentery, malaria; bladder inflammation caused by Candida fungi and gonococci, prostate inflammation; physical, nervous, and sexual asthenia; enlarged lymph nodes; low blood pressure; rheumatism, arthritis, rheumatic polyarthritis; psoriasis, aphtha, mycosis.

Main components: carvacrol, alpha-gamma-terpenes, thymol, p-zymene, beta-caryophyllene, alpha-humulene, linalool, damascenine.

Contraindications, side effects: caution recommended when using externally (very localized); caustic effect on skin and mucous membranes.

SOUTHERNWOOD (LAD'S LOVE):
Artemisia abrotanum (wp)—Asteraceae/Compositae
Properties: stimulates appetite, strengthening; sudorific; vermifuge; stimulates menstruation.
Contraindications, side effects: toxic in high doses.

SPIRAEA:
Spiraea ulmaria (fl)—Rosaceae
The essential oil is acquired through synergistic co-distillation.
Properties: Anti-rheumatic and diuretic (helps eliminate urine, uric acid, and chloride); anti-inflammatory; sudorific and astringent; against water collection in tissue; against stones in kidneys and bladder; against diarrhea; against cellulitis.

SPRUCE, BLACK:
Picea mariana Miller, Prel. Britt., Sterns, Pogg (n)—Abietaceae/Pinaceae
Properties: anti-spasmodic; against infection, mycosis, and parasites; germicide for the air; anti-inflammatory; general tonic; strengthens nerves.
Indications: bronchitis; asthenia; weakened immune system; muscle rheumatism; enteritis (intestinal catarrh) caused by fungi and parasites.
Main components: alpha-beta-pinene, 1-bornyl acetate, delta-3-carene, camphene, 1-alpha-phellandrene.
Contraindications, side effects: none known for normal dosages.

SPRUCE, RED OR COMMON SPRUCE:
Picea abies L., Karsten syn. Picea excelsa Link (n)—Abietaceae/Pinaceae
Properties: general antiseptic, especially for respiratory tract; against colds; against rheumatism; tonic; general stimulant.
Indications: acute and chronic bronchitis, sinusitis, colds; bladder inflammation; rheumatism, arthrosis; asthenia.
Main components: limonene, alpha-beta-pinene, camphene, bornyl acetate, myrcene, beta-phellandrene, Borneo Camphor, alpha-humulene.
Contraindications, side effects: none known for normal dosage; can irritate epidermis or mucous membranes if used undiluted.

SPRUCE, SITKA:
Epicea de Sitka, Picea sitchensis Bongard/Carr. (n)—Abietaceae/ Pinaceae

Properties: against infection, antibacterial; relieves coughs, expectorant, against colds; antifungal, against parasites; strengthening and stimulating; promotes wound healing and scar formation, germicide for the air.

Indications: bronchitis, sinusitis, influenza; infections of uro-genital systems; bladder inflammations caused by colibacteria; asthenia; rheumatism, muscle pain; skin ailments, mycosis; air disinfection.

Main components: myrcene, piperitone, 1-8-cineole, beta-phellandrene, limonene, isoamyl-isovalerate, isopentyl-isovalerate, alpha-beta-pinene.

Contraindications, side effects: use should be avoided by pregnant women and children.

ST. JOHN'S WORT:
Hypericum perforatum L . (wpm + fl)—Hypericaceae

Properties: general anti-inflammatory, especially for the mucous membranes; anti-spasmodic, against shock, hemostatic, antiseptic; stimulates the spleen.

Indications: inflammatory and post-traumatic processes; testicle inflammation; inflamed and spasmodic entercolitis; sprains, hemorrhage, stomach ulcers, nephritis, weakness of the spleen.

Main components: alpha-pinene, cadinene, hypericine, beta-caryophyllene, germacrene, 2-methyl octane, dodecanol.

Contraindications, side effects: persons subject to allergies should avoid external use.

SWEET CLOVER:
Melilotus officinalis (fl)—Fabaceae/Pipilionaceae
The essential oil is acquired through synergistic co-distillation.

Properties: Sedative and soporific; diuretic, antiseptic for urinary tract; anti-coagulant; for circulatory disorders.

SWEET FLAG:
Acorus calamus L. (r)—Araceae

Properties: diuretic, sudorific, stimulates appetite, strengthens stomach, promotes digestion, tonic, anti-spasmodic; anti-inflammatory for stomach and kidney area.

Indications: bladder inflammation; inflammation of stomach mucous membranes, digestive complaints, flatulence, stomach-intestinal-cramps; low blood pressure.

Main components: beta-azarone, d-alpha-pinene, camphene, cineole, camphor.

Contraindications, side effects: do not use over a longer period of time.

Sweet Gum, Oriental:

Liquidambar orientalis Mill., L. styracifluum L. (r)—Hamamelidaceae

Properties: anti-spasmodic, analgesic, relieves coughs; derivant, diuretic, dehydrating; against parasites.

Indications: bronchial colds, pneumonia, coughing, all states of cramping; ulcerated varicose veins, wounds, atonic wounds, abscess, frostbite, skin parasites (lice, mites).

Main components: cinnamic acid, styracine, cinnamethyl ether, vaniline, styral (cinnameine, storesinol, styrene).

Contraindications, side effects: none known for normal dosage.

Tagetes:

Tagetes minutus L., T. glanduliferus Schrank (wp + fl)—Asteraceae

Properties: against infection, antifungal, vermifuge; expectorant, against colds; promotes menstruation.

Indications: bronchial colds, sinusitis; enterocolitis caused by parasites, worm ailments, Candida mycosis; amenorrhea.

Main components: tagetone, cis- and trans-beta-ocimene, carvone, linalool, linalyl acetate.

Contraindications, side effects: use should be avoided by children and pregnant women due to ketone toxicity; caution when used externally because of photosensitizing.

Tangerine Hybrida:

Citrus retiulata Blanco hybrida (p)—Rutaceae

Properties: sedative, analgesic, relaxant, anti-spasmodic; promotes digestion, promotes bile production and drainage of gallbladder; stimulates circulation; antiseptic, fungicidal.

Indications: insomnia, neurasthenia, anxiety, cardiovascular erethism; digestive complaints, aerophagy, stomach pain; mycosis.

Main components: limonene, linalool, cumarine, furocumarine.

Contraindications, side effects: photosensitizing when applied externally.

TANSY:
Tanacetum balsamita L., Balsamita suavolens Pers. (wp)—Compositae
Properties: antibacterial and antiviral, antifungal, against parasites; expectorant; against hemorrhage (externally applied); anti-inflammatory; regenerates the skin and promotes wound healing; vermifuge.

Indications: bronchitis, sinusitis, colds; stomatitis, inflamed diarrhea, bladder and urethra inflammation; intestinal parasites; skin ailments, mycosis, wounds.

Main components: carvone, alpha-thujone, perille aldehyde, 1-8-cineole.

Contraindications, side effects: use should be avoided by children and pregnant women due to ketone toxicity; be certain to use low dosage for internal use.

TANSY, ANNUAL:
Tanacetum annuum L. (wp)—Asteraceae/Compositae
Properties: strong anti-inflammatory, anti-histamine; sedative, analgesic; reduces blood pressure (anti-leukemic); strengthens veins.

Indications: asthma, emphysema; skin inflammation, skin allergy; arythmia, little ruptured arteries; neuritis, sciatica, muscle rheumatism, arthritis; high blood pressure, venous stasis, varicose veins.

Main components: limonene, chamazulene.

Contraindications, side effects: none known for normal dosage; it has an endocrine effect in certain women (according to P. Franchomme and D. Pénoel).

TANSY, COMMON:
Tanacetum vulgare L., chrysanthemum tanacetum Karsch (wp)—Asteraceae/ Compositae
Properties: strengthening; anti-spasmodic; febrifuge; promotes menstruation; vermifuge.

Indications: intestinal worms and parasites, ailments due to worms; amenorrhea.

Main components: tanacetone = (beta-thujone), 1-camphor, borneol.

Contraindications, side effects: absolutely avoid use by pregnant women and children; generally not to be used regularly due to the ketone toxicity.

TARRAGON:
Artemisia dracunculus L. (wp)—Asteraceae/Compositae
Properties: generally stimulating, promotes digestion, stomachic; diuretic, anti-spasmodic; against rheumatism; promotes menstruation; vermifuge, antiviral; "anti-carcinogenic."

Indications: aerophagy, hiccups, inflamed and spasmodic colitis, constipation; neuromuscular cramps, spasmophilia, vegetative dystonia; painful and irregular menstruation, premenstrual syndrome;, viral diseases; kidney inflammation; sciatica; intestinal parasites.
Main components: methyl chavicol, estragol, zymene, linayl acetate.
Contraindications, side effects: none known for normal dosages.

TEA TREE:

Melaleuca alternifolia Maiden (l)—Myrtaceae
Properties: general disinfectant with broad spectrum, antibacterial, antimicrobial, antiviral, antifungal, against parasites; stimulates immune system; tonic for circulation and nerves; anti-inflammatory; protects against radiation damage.
Indications: infectious processes of all kinds; otitis, bronchitis, rhinopharyngitis, gum inflammation, tooth abscess, aphtha, pyorrhea (infection of the gums), stomatitis; infectious, viral, and parasitic enterocolitis; infection and congestive conditions of female organs; general and nervous asthenia; sensitivity to cold; cardiac insufficiency; burns due to radiation therapy (preventive); preparation for operative intervention with narcotics; Candida ailments, mycosis.
Main components: terpineol-4, alpha-gamma-terpinene, d-alpha-pinene, p-cymene, cineole, cadinene, viridiflorene, viridiflorol.
Contraindications, side effects: none known for normal dosage.

TEA TREE, LEMON:

Leptospermum petersoni L. citratum Chall. (l)—Myrtaceae
Properties: analgesic, anodyne, promotes digestion, anti-inflammatory.
Indications: neurasthenia, anxiety, depression; slow or difficult digestion, colitis, spasmic entercolitis.
Main components: geranial, neral, citronellal.
Contraindications, side effects: none known for normal dosage.

TURPENTINE:

Pinus pinaster Sol. (w + r)—Abietaceae/Pinaceae
Properties: antiseptic, thins secretion of windpipe and bronchial tract, relieves coughs, antiseptic for respiratory and urinary tract; dissolves gallstones; against rheumatism, pain remedy for rheumatism; vermifuge.
Indications: chronic bronchitis, colds, sinusitis, infection of the urinary tract and the kidneys, bladder inflammation, urethra inflammation, gallstone difficulties, edema, pyelitis, rheumatic neuralgia, rheumatism, gout;

intestinal parasites (tapeworm); for accidental intake of phosphorus (according to J. Valnet).

Main components: alpha-beta-pinene, dipentine, d-limonene.

Contraindications, side effects: can be used in very weak doses internally, with the exception of aerosol treatment and inhalation. Can irritate when used externally (possible skin allergies). Cannot be combined with any oxidants.

Thuja or Tree of Life:

Thuja occidentalis L. (l)—Cupressaceae

Properties: against infections of respiratory and urinary tract; against colds, expectorant; derivant, diuretic, and analgesic for urinary tract; against allergies; "anti-carcinogenic;" promotes wound healing and scar formation; antiviral, against virulent illness.

Indications: bronchial catarrh and viral bronchitis; bladder inflammation, enlarged prostate, pelvic congestion, herpes labialis; rheumatism; tumors, wounds, scars, warts, condyloma, polyps, papilloma, shingles, adenoids.

Main components: thujone, isothujone, fenchone, bornyl acetate, occidentalol, sabinene.

Contraindications, side effects: completely avoid for children and pregnant women due to the neurotoxic and abortive effect of the ketone content.

Thyme Varieties:

The variety of "Thymus vulgaris," our garden thyme, is a Mediterranean plant of the labiate family, which shows a remarkable chemical variety, especially the type grown in Provence. There are three basic groups of chemotypes:

1. Thymes of the "alcohol chemotype" (linalool, geraniol, alpha-terpineol, thujanol-4) called "mild thyme" or, as the distillers call it, "yellow thyme." Its essential oil is not aggressive and does not cause any oxidation of the distillation container (made of iron) by changing its color.
2. Thymes of the "monoterpene chemotyope" (paracymene).
3. Thymes of the "phenol chemotype" (thymol, carvacrol), which the distillers call "strong thyme"
   • or "red thyme" because of its thymols since the essential oil has a caustic effect; it turns the yellow color of the essential oil red

and causes the iron content of the distillation container's metal to oxidize;

- or "black thyme" because of its carvacrols since this is even more caustic and causes the original yellow of the essential oil to oxidize black.

This phenomena of oxidation is eliminated by using distillation containers made of rust-free steel.

THYME, MILD PROVENCE *(geraniol chemotype):*
Thymus vulgaris L. (wp + fl)—Labiatae

Properties: against infection and microbes, strong anti-bacterial effect, antiviral and antifungal; general strengthening and stimulant, especially for brain, heart, and uterus.

Indications: physical and mental asthenia; inflammation of mucous membranes of mouth and nose, bronchitis, otitis, sinusitis; bacterial enterocolitis caused by coli bacteria, viruses, and parasites; cardiac insufficiency, inflammations of urethra, bladder, vagina, cervix, and ovarian tubes; eases birth; shingles, acne, eczema, skin ailments, wounds, mycosis.

Main components: geraniol, myrcenol, geranyl acetate.

Contraindications, side effects: none known for normal dosage.

THYME, MILD PROVENCE *(linalool chemotype):*
Thymus vulgaris L. (wp + fl)—Labiatae

Properties: against infection, antimicrobial, antibacterial, antiviral, and antifungal; vermifuge; general tonic; strengthens immune system; stimulates central nervous system, nerve reflexes, and uterus; anti-spasmodic, aphrodisiac.

Indications: bronchitis, pneumonia, pleurisy, tuberculosis; gastritis, stomatitis; bacterial, viral, and Candida-caused entercolitis; parasite-caused colitis; Candida-caused vaginal and bladder inflammation; uterine and ovarian tube inflammation caused by staphylococci; viral prostate inflammation, kidney tuberculosis; agitation, spasmophilia, nervous exhaustion; muscle rheumatism; skin ailments, psoriasis, warts.

Main components: linalool, linyl acetate, terpinene, p-cymene, thymol.

Contraindications, side effects: none known for normal dosage.

THYME, MILD PROVENCE (paramcymene chemotype):
Thymus vulgaris L. (wp + fl)—Labiatae
Properties: strengthening, general stimulant, slight disinfectant effect, germicide for the air; analgesic, especially for transcutaneous administration.
Indications: asthenia, exhaustion; disinfectant for the air; arthrosis, rheumatism, muscle rheumatism.
Main components: p-cymene, gamma-terpinene, thymol.
Contraindications, side effects: use internally only in weak dosage; can irritate sensitive skin when used externally (dilute the essential oil 10 to20%, even to 50% with plant oil).

THYME, MILD PROVENCE (thujanol-4 chemotype):
Thymus vulgaris L.(wp + fl)—Labiatae
Properties: against infection, antibacterial, strong anti-viral effect; stimulates immune system; stimulates circulation, gallbladder, and digestion; stimulating and balancing for the nerves (central nervous system, medulla oblongata, and cerebellum); against diabetes.
Indications: influenza, otitis, bronchitis, sinusitis, rhinopharyngitis, tonsil inflammation; slow or difficult digestion, flatulence, stomatitis, inflamed or viral enterocolitis, liver insufficiency, diabetes; bladder inflammation, vulva inflammation, vaginitis, cervical inflammation; insufficient urination, prostate inflammation, condyloma of the genitals; arthrosis, tendonitis; nervous disturbances, neurasthenia, insomnia of nervous origin, asthenia; skin ailments, skin inflammation.
Main components: thujanol-4, myrcenol, myrcenyl acetate, linalool, myrcene, gamma-terpinene.
Contraindications, side effects: none known for normal dosage.

THYME, MILD (alpha-terpineol chemotype):
Thymus vulgaris L.
Is currently being researched and will be presented in detail in a later edition.

THYME, MILD SPANISH EUCALYPTOLE (chemotype 1-8-cineole):
Thymus membranaceus (wp + fl)—Labiatae
Properties: against infection, antibacterial, antimicrobial, and antifungal; expectorant, against colds, relieves coughs; strengthening, stimulates circulation.

Indications: bronchitis, otitis, sinusitis, rhinopharyngitis; intestinal infections, Candida mycosis of uro-genital system; asthenia; circulatory disturbances.

Main components: 1-8-cineole, camphor, camphene, alpha-beta-pinene, myrcene, sabinene, borneol.

Contraindications, side effects: do not use for babies.

THYME, STRONG PROVENCE *(carvacrol chemotype):*
Thymus vulgaris L. (wp + fl)—Labiatac

Properties: important disinfectant with broad spectrum; antimicrobial, antibacterial, antiviral, antifungal, and against parasites; general physical and mental strengthening and stimulation, especially for circulation; raises blood pressure; analgesic; vermifuge.

Indications: infections in throat-nose-ear area, respiratory tract, stomach-intestinal tract, urogenital system; asthenia, exhaustion, atony of blood circulation; rheumatism, arthritis; intestinal parasites, mycosis.

Main components: carvacrol, p-cymene, thymol, gamma-terpinene.

Contraindications, side effects: when applied externally, irritates the skin and mucous membranes because of phenol content (use the essential oil diluted with 5 to 10% plant oil).

THYME, STRONG PROVENCE *(thymol chemotype):*
Thymus vulgaris L. (wp + fl)—Labiatae

Properties: important disinfectant; antimicrobial, antibacterial, antiviral, and antifungal; physically and emotionally stimulating and strengthening; stimulates circulation (particularly capillary vessels); promotes digestion; relieves coughs, expectorant; diuretic, stimulates bile production and drainage of gallbladder; raises blood pressure; vermifuge.

Indications: infections in throat-nose-ear area, respiratory tract, stomach-intestinal tract, and uro-genital system; asthenia, exhaustion, atony of the circulation and the digestion, anemia; joint and muscle rheumatism, gout; intestinal parasites, mycosis, skin ailments.

Main components: thymol, p-cymene, gamma-terpinene, carvacrol.

Contraindications, side effects: irritates the skin and mucous membranes when applied externally due to phenol content (use the essential oil diluted 5 to 10% with plant oil).

THYME, STRONG SPANISH OR ZYGIS THYME *(thymol chemotype):*
Thymus zygis ssp. sylvestris (wp + fl)—Labiatae

The Spanish zygis thymes have more chemotypes:

Aside from the *Thymus cygis ssp. sylvestris* with thymol, there is *Thymus zygis gracilis* with paracymene thymol and *Thymus cygis cygis* with terpenyl acetate.

Properties: against infection, antimicrobial, antibacterial and antiviral; analgesic; general physical and mental strengthening and stimulation, especially circulation and digestion.

Indications: infections in throat-nose-ear area; bronchitis, angina, otitis, sinusitis; infections of stomach-intestinal tract and uro-genital system; rheumatism, arthrosis; asthenia, atony of the circulation and digestion.

Main components: thymol, p-cymene, 1-8-cineole, gamma-terpinene, alpha-pinene, camphene, borneol, linalool.

Contraindications, side effects: not for use by babies, small children, or pregnant women; irritates the skin and mucous membranes when used undiluted.

THYME, WILD:

Thymus serpyllum L. (wp)—Lamiaceae/Labiatae

Properties: against infection, antibacterial, antiviral, and antifungal; general stimulant and strengthening, especially for respiratory tract; against cough irritation, expectorant; promotes bile production and drainage of gallbladder; promotes digestion, carminative; anti-spasmodic, analgesic, against rheumatism; against parasites and worms.

Indications: influenza, bronchitis, coughing, whooping cough, asthma, emphysema, tuberculosis; stomach-intestinal infections, infectious enterocolitis, stomach pain, dyspepsia, flatulence; bladder inflammation, infection of urinary tract; rheumatism, sciatica, lumbago; infectious skin inflammation, impetigo, abscess, panaritium (pus-inflammed fingers), wounds.

Main components: thymol, carvacrol, p-cymene, linalool, geraniol, borneol, alpha-pinene, gamma-terpinene.

Contraindications, side effects: none for normal dosage; however, due to the phenol content of about 30%, is caustic and irritating to the mucous membranes.

THYME, WILD LEMON:

Thymus serpyllum ssp. praecox, T. citriodorus Schreb. (wp + fl) = Lamiaceae/Labiatae

Properties: general stimulant; antimicrobial, antibacterial, antiviral, and antifungal; sedative for nerves, anti-inflammatory.

Indications: physical and mental asthenia; infection in throat-nose-ear area, stomach-intestinal tract. and uro-genital system; mouth and gum infection, sinusitis, otitis, bronchitis, bacterial and viral enteritis; urethra inflammation, bladder inflammation, and vaginitis; acne, eczema, mycosis.

Main components: geraniol, geranial, nerale, nerol, terpinene-4-ol.

Contraindications, side effects: none known for normal dosage; can be irritating to the skin when applied externally, due to the citral content.

TOLU BALSAM:

Myroxylon toluiferum, Toluifera balsamum

(r)—Fabaceae/Papilionaceae

Properties: antiseptic for respiratory tract, relieves coughs, expectorant; antiseptic for urinary tract; for skin ailments.

Indications: bronchial catarrh and chronic bronchitis, coughing, pneumonia, tuberculosis; bladder inflammation, urethra inflammation, prostate inflammation.

Main components: styrene and beta-caryophyllene, benzyl alcohol and benzyl acid, cinnamic acid, cinnamic alcohol.

Contraindications, side effects: irritation possible when used externally over longer period of time.

TURMERIC:

Curcuma domestica C. longa L., Curcuma xanthorriza (r)—Zingiberaceae

Properties: bactericide, stimulant for liver and gallbladder; promotes bile production and drainage of gallbladder, against gallstones; lowers cholesterol; against cellulitis.

Indications: colitis; cellulitis; worm ailments; liver-gallbladder insufficiency; high cholesterol level; skin ailments; rheumatism.

Main components: turmerol, turmerone, curcumone, cineole, camphene, d-alpha-pinene.

Contraindications, side effects: internal use, particularly by children and pregnant women, should be avoided.

VALERIAN:

Valeriana officinalis (r)—Valerianaceae

Properties: balancing effect on nerves, psyche, and heart; anti-spasmodic, sedative, hypothermic.

Indications: psychological and sensory overexcitation; shaking (Parkinson's disease), neurasthenia, insomnia, tachycardia, spasmophilia, fever, hot flashes, malaria, nervous asthma.

Main components: isovalerian-acid, bornyl-isovalerate, a-terpeneol, kessyl-alcohol, kessyl-acetate, a-pinene, camphene, limonene, borneol, camphor.

Contraindications, side effects: none known for normal doses, toxic in higher doses. Can lead to habit with longer use.

VERBENA OR LEMON STALK:

Lippia citriodora H.B. and Kuntze (l)—Verbenaceae

Properties: sedative and analgesic; anti-inflammatory, soothing, febrifuge; stimulates nerves and gonads (testicles, ovaries); dissolves stones; against infections.

Indications: exhaustion and nervous states of depression, insomnia, stress, anxiety; multiple sclerosis; insufficiency of liver, gallbladder, and pancreas; digestive complaints, diarrhea, malaria, amoebic dysentery (cysts caused by amoebas), Morbus Crohn (rectal inflammation); gallbladder inflammation, diabetes, bladder inflammation, stone build-up in urinary tract; cardiac insufficiency; tachycardia, coronaritis; Hodgkinson's disease; overexertion of the eyes; asthma; rheumatism; psoriasis.

Main components: citral, geranial, neral, limonene, beta-caryopyllene, curcumene, a-farnesene, a-terpineol, nerolidol, neryl acetate, 1-8-cineole.

Contraindications, side effects: none known for normal dosage; slightly irritating and photosensitizing when applied externally.

VETIVER:

Vetiveria zizanoides Stapf. V. muricata Griseb. Andropogon muriatus Retz., A. squarrosus Hack. (r)—Poaceae

Properties: general strengthening and stimulating (glandular system, circulation); stimulates immune system; against rheumatism; promotes menstruation; against parasites; repels insects; germicide for the air.

Indications: mental exhaustion; circulatory weakness, coronaritis; liver-pancreas insufficiency; immune depression; rheumatism; arthrosis; amenorrhea, infrequent menstruation; urticaria; skin parasites, skin care; room disinfectant.

Main components: vetiverol, vetivene, a-b-vetivone, vetivenyl acetate, vetiverone, cadinene.

Contraindications, side effects: should not be used by babies and pregnant women.

VIOLET, AROMATIC:

Viola odorata (wp)—Violaceae

The essential oil is acquired through synergistic co-distillation.

Properties: anti-inflammatory for digestive and urinary tract; emollient, sudorific, relieves coughs.

Visnaga:

(Khella) Ammi visnaga L. (wp + s)—Apiaceae/Umbelliferae

Properties: dilates coronary vessels; anti-coagulant, anti-asthmatic, against intestinal infection.

Indications: coronary insufficiencies, arteriosclerosis; asthma, kidney and gallbladder colic; colitis.

Main components: visnadine, kelline, kellol, linalool.

Contraindications, side effects: photosensitizing when applied externally.

WINTERGREEN:

Gaultheria fragrantissima Wall. (l)—Myrtaceae

Properties: anti-spasmodic, anti-inflammatory, expansion of the vessels, analgesic.

Indications: arthritis, rheumatism, rheumatic polyarthritis; tendonitis, cramps; liver insufficiency; high blood pressure, headache, inflammation of coronary vessels; skin allergies.

Contraindications, side effects: none known for normal dosage.

WINTERGREEN OR CREEPING GAULTHERIA:

Gaultheria procumbens L. (l)—Ericaceae

Wintergreen is relatively rare on the market and very frequently imitated. It has practically the same composition as *black birch (Betula lenta)* or *yellow birch (Betula alleganiensis)*, which means between 95 and 99% methyl salizylate.

Properties: anti-inflammatory, analgesic, anti-spasmodic; stimulates the liver, diuretic, blood purifier; against rheumatism, vessel expanding.

Indications: rheumatism, arthrosis, arthritis, rheumatic polyarthritis, muscle rheumatism, tendonitis, cramps; liver insufficiency; high blood pressure; migraine caused by liver and circulation disturbances; coronaritis; shingles.

Main components: methyl salizylate—98%.

Contraindications, side effects: none known for normal dosage.

WORMWOOD:
Artemisia absinthium L. (wp + fl)—Asteraceae
Properties: stimulates appetite, strengthens digestion, bitter tonic; promotes menstruation (in case of amenorrhea); vermifuge.
Main components: alpha- and beta-thujone, absinthiine, palmitinic acid, isovalerianic acid.
Contraindications, side effects: it is dangerous to overdose when using internally because of abortive and neurotoxic effect.

YLANG-YLANG VARIETIES:
The properties of the essential oils from ylang-ylang change depending on the length of distillation. The first distillation phase is the "head of the distillation," where the most volatile essential oil yields the quality "Ylang extra," highly prized by perfumeries. Afterwards come the qualities "Ylang 1, 2, 3, 4" and so forth, the "body" or "tail" of the essential oil with its heavier portions. A decrease in alcohol and acetate content occurs, as well as an increase in sesquiterpene. On the therapeutic level, as for all essential oils we naturally prefer the pure essence ylang oil "complete."

YLANG-YLANG "EXTRA":
Cananga odorata Lamarck (fl)—Anonaceae
Properties: anti-spasmodic, anti-inflammatory; balancing, regulating, and stimulating for the heart; lowers blood pressure, dampens excitation of reflexes; against infection of respiratory tract and genitalia; sexual stimulant.
Indications: cardiac insufficiency, tachycardia, high blood pressure, spasmophilia; infection of respiratory tract and genitalia; sexual asthenia, frigidity, impotence; skin and hair care.
Main components: germacrene, benzyl benzoate, linalool, cadinene-alpha-farnesene, beta-caryophyllene, anisol menthyl, benzyl benzoate, cinnamyl acetate.
Contraindications, side effects: none known for normal dosage.

YLANG-YLANG "COMPLETE":
Cananga odorata genuina Lamrck (fl)—Anonaceae
Properties: anti-spasmodic, anti-inflammatory; balancing, regulating, and stimulating for the heart; lowers blood pressure, dampens excitation of reflexes; against infection of respiratory tract and genitalia; general stimulant and strengthening remedy; sexual stimulant; germicide for the air.

154

Indications: cardiac insufficiency, tachycardia, high blood pressure, spasmophilia; infection of respiratory tract and genitalia; physical, mental, and sexual asthenia; frigidity, impotence; skin and hair care; air freshening.
Main components: germacrene (27%), beta-caryophyllene, cadinene-farnesene, geranyl acetate, linalool, benzyl benzoate, humulene-cadinene.
Contraindications, side effects: none known for normal dosage.

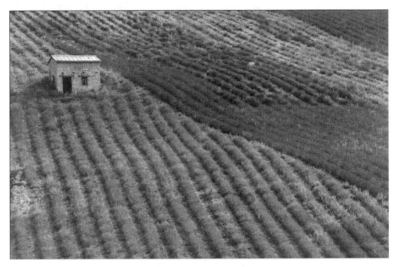

Lavender field in Provence

Table of Essential Oils

(Divided into practical criteria for the consumer)

The essential oils which have been previously discussed have been divided into various categories according to their practical value, therapeutic effect, and cost.

Essences which are frequently used can be found in columns 1, 2, and 3.

- The first column lists 25 very commonly used essential oils which can be defined as the basic essential oils.

These were the decisive characteristics for listing essential oils in this category:

- Plants, either wild or cultivated, which are major sources of essential oil.
- Simple techniques for acquisition of essential oil through distillation.
- A good to fair yield of essential oil.
- Frequent and convenient use in therapy.
- Widely available and reasonably priced.

These 25 essential oils form the actual basis of an aromatic first-aid kit. They cover a great majority of therapeutic and hygiene applications.

- Column 2 lists more common essential oils which broaden the range of those listed in column 1. In part, these are varieties whose properties are quite specific.
- Column 3 lists other fairly common essential oils which are also used frequently. They are important due to their properties, but have a low yield and correspondingly high cost.
- Columns 4 and 5 list rare and expensive essential oils. They come from plants with a minor content of essential oil and have very limited availability. Although some oleoresins are not very expensive, they are still difficult to find. From a therapeutic viewpoint, a number of essential oils from this list are very interesting but should only be used on the advice of a naturopath or aromatherapist. This category also includes some precious perfume fragrances.
- Similar to columns 4 and 5, column 6 lists those essential oils which are used infrequently, but are inexpensive. These are extracted from plants and highly aromatic trees.

Table

The division of the essential oils into the various categories presented on this table is not rigid. In column 1, for example, a few of the essential oils could be omitted and others added without being incorrect. However, this classification is based upon a solid foundation and should be used as a guide.

In order to create a link between this table and the therapeutic index, we have summarized the above information into three points:

1. The 25 very common essential oils listed in column 1 form a good basis from which to prepare your own treatment and body-care products. One approach would be to use this list as a basis when consulting the therapeutic index. Only the basic essences would then be considered for use in treatment.
2. Columns 2 and 3 offer a selection of essential oils for use by well-informed and experienced users such naturopaths, reflexologists, massage therapists, etc. It is also possible to limit the selection from the therapeutic index to the essential oils from these first 3 columns.
3. Use of the essential oils from the columns 4, 5, and 6 should be limited to therapists. Also keep in mind that the rare and expensive essential oils in the columns 3, 4, and 5 are very frequently adulterated. In your own interest as a consumer, be sure to demand a guarantee of quality. This promotes a consciousness of quality and promotes the production and sale of essential oils which are qualitatively flawless.

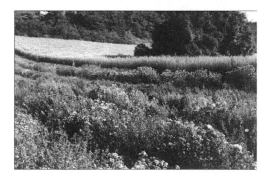

Test plots

Commonly Used Essential Oils

1. Very Common	2. Common	3. Fairly Common But Expensive
Anise	Anise, Chinese ▲	Angelica ▲
Basil	Bergamot	Carrot
Birch	Boldo	Celery
Cajeput	Borneo Camphor ▲	Chamomile, Roman
Chamomile, (A. mixta)	Cade	Chamomile, True or
Clove ▲	Caraway ▲	German
Eucalyptus globulus	Cedar	Cinnamon, Ceylon ▲
Geranium	Cinnamon (leaf)	Melissa
Juniper	Citronella	Cumin
Lavandin	Coriander	Ginger
Lavender, True	Eucalyptus camald.	Incense
Lemon	Eucalyptus citriodora	Marjoram (O. maior)
Marjoram (T. mastich.)	Eucalyptus radiata	Myrrh
Niaouli	Fennel ▲	Parsley ▲
Orange	Grapefruit	Ravensara
Origanum, Span. ▲	Hyssop (H. officinalis) ▲	Sage, Clary
Peppermint ▲	Laurel	Sandalwood ▲
Pine (P. silvestr.)	Lavender, Spike	Spiraea
Rosemary ▲	Lemongrass	St. John's Wort
Sage, (S. offic.) ▲	Mandarin	Tarragon
Savory ▲	Mint, Wood ▲	Valerian ▲
Thyme, Mild	Myrtle	Verbena
Thyme, Strong ▲	Nutmeg ▲	
Thyme, Wild	Orange, Bitter	
Turpentine ▲	Palmarosa	
	Patchouli	
	Pennyroyal ▲	
	Rosewood	
	Sassafras	
	Sweet Flag	
	Thuja ▲	
	Ylang-Ylang	

Rarely Used Essential Oils

4. Rare and Expensive		5. Rarely Used and Inexpensive
Benzoin	Peru Balsam	Balsam, Canada
Boxwood	Rose	Bay
Buchu	Santolina	Copaiba Balsam
Cardamom	Southernwood ▲	Corkwood
Cinnamon, China ▲	Sweet Clover	Dill
Cubeb	Sweet Gum, Oriental	Elemi
Curcuma	Tansy ▲	Fir
Elder	Tolu Balsam ▲	Guajac
Elecampane	Violet	Gurjun
Everlasting gymnoc.	Visnaga	Lime, Sweet
Everlasting Italian		Mugwort ▲
Galbanum		Petitgrain, Bitter Orange
Garlic ▲		Petitgrain, Lemon
Gentian		Pine:
Goldenrod		– Beach Pine
Hawthorne		– Black Pine
Horseradish		– Siberian Pine
Hyssop, Wild ▲		Rue ▲
Inula		Savin ▲
Iris		Vetiver
Labdanum		Wintergreen ▲
Lantana		
Larch		
Linden		
Linden Sapwood		
Lovage		
Mace		
Mimosa		
Mustard		
Neroli		
Onion		
Origanum, Common ▲		
Pepper		

Note: There are application restrictions for essences marked with ▲.
Please look up the respective entry in Chapter VII.

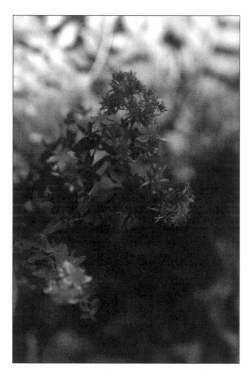

St. John's Wort

Chapter VIII

Therapeutic Index

Preliminary Remarks

Most diseases are caused by a lack of respect for biological laws and the natural and cosmic order, of which we are a part. This means that any therapy, including treatment with natural therapies, must be supported and reinforced by a healthy lifestyle: light, wholesome food; breathing exercises on a regular basis; physical and mental training (relaxation, positive thinking, and energizing, especially in the open countryside).

Thinking is a form of energy, which is either negative or positive according the content we give our thoughts. Both tradition and modern research agree that the majority of dysfunctions and diseases have their origin within the psyche. This especially effects the immune system. A positive state of body, mind, and soul is therefore a fundamental prerequisite for restoring health.

In many ways, we create our own diseases through bad habits and living conditions. Conversely, we have the power to create good habits and activate the healing powers which are within us (and not outside us). Remember that the healing comes from nature itself—any types therapies and drugs only assist in this process.

The following therapeutic index is not intended to replace consultation with doctors, naturopaths, or aromatherapists. A doctor should definitely be consulted for serious or chronic cases. This also applies when there is doubt regarding the cause or diagnosis of an ailment.

Phytotherapy and aromatherapy are natural types of therapy. Like every other useful thing, however, there can also be dangers involved. When used incorrectly and without the necessary knowledge, they can also have undesirable effects.

We would like to again draw your attention to the basic rules and dosage directions for treatments with essential oils. See chapters V and VI of this book, as well as the reference works mentioned in the bibliography.

Treatment with essential oils (aromatherapy) combines very well with phytotherapy (herb teas, tinctures, powders, etc.), oligotherapy, and many other natural forms of therapy. In most cases, it can also provide effective support for an allopathic course of treatment.

In the following therapeutic index, the essential oils recommended can either be used internally or externally. It is specifically state if they are meant for external use only.

Instructions for Use of Therapeutic Index

1. First use the index to look up the essential oils related to your main symptom and make a list of them.
2. Make a list of the appropriate essential oils for your other weak points or secondary symptoms (such as high blood pressure, nervousness, insomnia, rheumatism, liver complaints, or digestive complaints) and check whether some of those already selected from the first list also appear on it. Select those essential oils which appear more than once on the lists. (See example in chapter V, pg. 61 ff).
3. Check the table at the end of chapter VII for the essential oils which are commonly used and therefore presumably available from your retailer.
4. Carefully read the instructions on how to make preparations:
   - For internal use: Chapter VI, pg. 70 ff
   - For external use: Chapter VI, pg. 74 ff
   - For use in cooking: Chapter VI, pg. 79
5. As already mentioned in the discussion of aromas and perfumes, it is important for you to use your sense of smell when selecting essential oils. It creates a direct connection between the aromas and what the body requires. When we experience a fragrance to be pleasant, it will contribute to our healing process. On the other hand, if we find the smell of a substance to be repulsive, we should avoid using it even in mixtures. More and more, aromatherapists are making allowances for their patients' reactions to certain fragrances.

Therapeutic Index

Abscess: *hot (acute infection with formation of pus):* Onion. *cold (slowly forming abscess without inflammation):* Cade, Camphor, Chamomile, Garlic, Juniper, Lavender, Lemon, Oriental Sweet Gum, Origanum, Sandalwood, Savory, Spike Lavender, Thyme, Wild Thyme.

Acne: Benzoin, Cajeput, Common Sage, Eucalyptus radiata, Juniper, Lavender, Lemon, Palmarosa, Patchouli, Petitgrain (Bitter Orange), Sandalwood.

Adenitis: See *Lymph Nodes, Swelling.*

Aerocoly: Agastache, Angelica, Bergamot, Chinese Anise, Tangerine.

Aerophagy (swallowing air, flatulence): Anise, Basil, Caraway, Cinnamon, Common Sage, Coriander, Fennel, Lemon, Marjoram, Mint varieties, Myrtle, Origanum, Savory, Tarragon, Thyme.

Aging, Premature: Birch, Borneol, Carrot, Chamomile, Clary Sage, Common Sage, Garlic, Horseradish, Juniper, Lavender, Lemon, Marjoram, Mints, Neroli, Nutmeg, Onion, Orange, Parsley, Rosemary, Savory, Thuja, Thyme.

Albumin: (in urine, result of kidney disorder): Canadian Erigeron, Juniper.

Allergies (harmful change of humoral terrain caused by external agent): Sanitize the terrain, non-toxic diet (see chapter IX), improvement of liver activity, blood purification. Achillea Ligustica, Bergamot, Birch, Boldo, Carrot, Chamomile, Common Sage, Gaultheria, Juniper, Laurel, Lavender, Lemon, Orange, Rosemary, Wintergreen.

Alopecia: See *Baldness.*

Amebic Dysentery: Cajeput leucadendron, Chamomile, Cinnamon, Elemi, Eucalyptus polybractea, Lemon Mint, Origanum, Savory, Verbena.

Amenorrhea: See *Periods.*

Anal Fistula: Lavender, Niaouli.

Anemia (reduction of number of red-blood corpuscles): Angelica, Basil, Carrot, Chamomile, Common Sage, Fennel, Goldenrod, Lemon, Orange, Parsley, Rosemary, Savory, Thyme, Wild Thyme.

Analgesic (relieves pain): Angelica, Anise, Basil, Borneo Camphor, Chamomile, Clove, Common Sage, Eucalyptus, Everlasting, Fennel, Gaultheria, Ginger, Juniper, Laurel, Lavandin, Marjoram, Mint, Nutmeg, Origanum, Ravensara, Rose Geranium, Sassafras, Savory, Tansy, Thyme, Wild Thyme.

Anorexia (loss of weight, causes often psychological): see under *Appetite, Loss of.*

Antiseptic (internal and external): most essential oils, but especially: Anise, Aspic, Bergamot, Borneo Camphor, Cade (externally), Cajeput, Caraway, Chamomile, Cinnamon, Clove, Eucalyptus, Garlic, Incense, Juniper, Lavender, Lemon, Mint, Niaouli, Origanum, Savory, Spike Lavender, Tea Tree, Thyme.

Anxiety (neuro-vegetative imbalance); Angelica, Anise, Basil, Cat Mint, Creeping Hyssop, Eucalyptus camaldulensis, Fennel, Incense, Lavender, Marjoram, Melissa, Neroli, Petitgrain (Combava), Tangerine, Thyme, Valerian, Verbena.

Aphony (loss of voice): Cypress, Lemon, Thyme.

Aphrodisiac (stimulates sexual desire): Anise, Borneo Camphor, Cedar, Cinnamon, Clary Sage, Clove, Ginger, Juniper, Mint, Neroli, Nutmeg, Pine, Rose, Rosemary, Sandalwood, Savory, Verbena, Ylang-Ylang.

Aphtha: Basil, Chamomile, Common Sage, Corkwood, Fennel, Lantana, Laurel, Lemon, Rose Geranium, Rose, Savory, Tea Tree, Wild Thyme.

Appetite, Loss of: Caraway, Carrot, Chamomile, Common Sage, Coriander, Fennel, Garlic, Ginger, Juniper, Lemon, Origanum, Tarragon.

Arrhythmia (irregularity of pulse): see Palpitations.

Arteriosclerosis (calcification of arteries and changes in vessel walls): Leek, Niaouli, Visnaga.

Arteritis (inflammation of arteries): Goldenrod, Lemongrass, Niaouli.

Arthritis, Arthrosis: See *Rheumatism.*

Asthenia (general weakness):
General: Angelica, Anise, Basil, Bupleurum, Calamint, Carrot, Chamomile, Cinnamon, Common Sage, Eucalyptus, Fennel, Ginger, Juniper, Lavender, Lemon, Mace, Marjoram, Melissa, Mint, Nutmeg, Parsley, Rosemary, Savory, Thyme, Vetiver, Wild Thyme.
Mental strain: Basil, Clove, Rosemary, Savory, Thyme.
Influenza: Cinnamon, Lemon, Common Sage, Thyme.
Weak nerves: Angelica, Basil, Melissa.
Sexual weakness: See *Impotency.*

Asthma: Angelica, Borneo Camphor, Cajeput, Carrot, Common Sage, Elecampane, Eucalyptus, Fennel, Garlic, Hyssop, Iris, Lantana, Lavender, Lemon, Marjoram, Melissa, Niaouli, Onion, Orange, Origanum, Parsley, Pennyroyal, Peppermint, Pine, Southernwood, St. John's Wort, Tansy annual, Tarragon, Thyme, Valerian, Verbena, Visnaga.
Nervous asthma: Angelica, Anise, Savory, Valerian. Antispasmodic effect.

Backache: Diagnosis. *For external use*: Birch, Borneol, Camphor, Chamomile, Peru Balsam, Vetiver, Wintergreen.

Bad Breath: Clarify the cause (liver, stomach, teeth). Anise, Cardamom, Chamomile, Coriander, Fennel, Lemon, Mints, Orange, Sweet Flag, Thyme, Wild Thyme.

Baldness: Cedar, Chamomile, Clary Sage, Common Sage, Lavender, Lemon, Rosemary, Thyme, Wild Thyme, Ylang-ylang.

Bedwetting (incontinence): Cypress, Juniper (berries). Remineralization.

Bile: *Insufficient production*: Anise, Boldo, Chamomile, Lavender, Rosemary. Pythotherapy: Chicory, Dandelion.
Not fluid enough: Boldo, Carrot, Lemon, Rosemary. Phytotherapy: Artichoke, Burdock, Chicory.
To promote elimination: Carrot, Pennyroyal. Phytotherapy: Combretum, Hemp Agrimony, Milfoil, Radish.

Birth, Facilitating: Clove, Mugwort, Nutmeg, Sage. Phytotherapy: Lady's Mantle.
Also see Uterus: stimulant.

Bladder Infection: Bay, Bergamot, Borneo Camphor, Buchu, Cajeput, Canada Balsam, Cat Mint, Cedar, Chamomile, Cinnamon, Clove, Copaiva Balsam, Coriander, Cubeb, Eucalyptus, Fir, Gurjun, Hyssop (Creeping), Inula, Juniper, Large-Leafed Basil, Lavender, Lemon, Mints, Myrrh, Myrtle, Niaouli, Origanum, Palmarosa, Parsley, Patchouli, Pepper, Peru Balsam, Pine, Rosemary (Cineol), Sandalwood, Sassafras, Savory, Spruce, Sweet Flag, Tea Tree, Thyme varieties, Tolu Balsam, Turpentine, Wild Thyme.

Bleeding: Consult doctor. Bergamot, Cinnamon, Cypress, Juniper, Lavender, Lemon, Rose Geranium, Spike Lavender, Thyme, Wild Thyme.

Blepharitis: See *Conjunctivitis*. Do not put any essential oils in the eyes! Treat with infusions.

Blood Pressure, High: Basil, Birch, Canadian Erigeron, Carrot, Eucalyptus citiodora, Garlic, Gaultheria, Hawthorn, Inula, Juniper, Lavender, Lemon, Marjoram, Melissa, Neroli, Niaouli, Nutmeg, Peppermint, Sassafras, Spike Lavender, Tansy (annual), Verbena, Wintergreen (creeping), Ylang-ylang.

Blood Pressure, Low: Cinnamon, Common Sage, Hawthorne, Hyssop, Peppermint, Rosemary, Thyme.

Blood Purification: Angelica, Birch, Borneo Camphor, Carrot, Chamomile, Common Sage, Cypress, Fennel, Gentian, Grapefruit, Juniper, Lavender, Lemon, Onion, Orange, Parsley, Peppermint, Rosemary, Sassafras, Savory, Sweet Flag, Thuja, Wild Thyme, Wintergreen.

165

Blood Thinning: Carrot, Lemon, Inula.

Boils (furunculosis): Non-toxic diet (see Chapter IX). Bergamot, Carrot, Chamomile, Cinnamon, Juniper, Lemon, Niaouli, Petitgrain (Bitter Orange), Sage, Sandalwood, Savory, Thyme.

Bones: See *Demineralization* and *Rickets*.

Breast-Feeding: *To stimulate milk flow*: Anis-Ravansara, Anise, Caraway, Common Sage, Cumin, Dill, Fennel, Laurel, Parsley, Peppermint, Verbena.

To stop lactation: Chervil, Common Sage, Laurel, Parsley, Peppermint, St. John's Wort.

Breasts: *Swelling*: Chervil, Cumin, Fennel, Mints, Parsley, Rose Geranium.

Inflammation (Mastitis): Parsley

Cracked nipples: Benzoin, Borneo Camphor, Carrot, Incense, Lemon, Onion, Peru Balsam, Sandalwood, Turpentine.

Bronchitis: Achillea Ligustica, Angelica, Basil (Eugenol), Cajeput, Calamint, Canada Balsam, Chinese Anise, Cinnamon, Common Sage, Copaiba balsam, Dill, Elecampane, Eucalyptus, Garlic, Hyssop, Inula, Iris, Lantana, Lemon, Lovage, Mint, Mustard, Niaouli, Origanum, Peru Balsam, Pine, Ravensara, Rosemary, Savory, Sitka Spruce, Southernwood, Tagetes, Tansy, Tea Tree, Thyme, Tolu Balsam.

Bulima: Usually has psychological causes. Angelica, Basil, Rosemary, Valerian.

Burns (first and second degree): Apply the following blend of essential oils undiluted (equal quantities of each): Chamomile, Common Sage, Eucalyptus, Lavender, Niaouli, Rose Geranium, Rosemary.

Burns from Radiation Therapy (preventive): Niaouli, Tea Tree.

Cancer (malignant tumors): Seek medical help. Change your diet and your lifestyle.

To support treatment and prevention, the following essential oils are recommended: Balsam Pine, Chervil, Clove, Common Sage, Cypress, Garlic, Hyssop, Juniper, Lovage, Onion, Parsley, Pennyroyal, Rose Geranium, Tarragon, Thuja, Wood Mint.

Capillaries, Fragile: Anise, Carrot, Celery, Grapefruit, Horseradish, Lemon, Orange, Origanum vulgaris, Rue, Thyme (strong), Thymol.

Cataract (gray): Seek medical help. Ginger, Larch, Fine Lavender (internally). Aromatic hydrolate: Ginger (externally).

Cellulite: See *Weight-Loss Diet*.

Chickenpox: see *Measles*.

Chills: Clarify cause. Cinnamon, Ginger, Nutmeg, Rosemary, Sage, Wild Thyme.

Chlorosis: Young women's anemia: Angelica, Carrot, Chamomile, Lavender, Pine, Rosemary, Thyme (mild), Wild Thyme. Also see Anemia.

Cholecystitis (inflammation of gallbladder): Also see *Gallbladder stones*. Boldo, Boxwood, Common Pine, Eucalyptus, Melissa, Mountain Pine, Orange, Peppermint, Rosemary, Thyme, Valerian, Verbena.

Cholera: Bush Rosemary, Ravensara.

Cholesterol, High: Angelica, Camphor, Carrot, Clary Sage, Curcuma, Everlasting italicum, Fennel, Lemon, Onion, Rosemary, Sage, Spanish Rosemary, Thyme, Verbena.

Circulation, Poor: Agastache, Anise, Basil (large-leafed), Bay, Birch, Bitter Orange, Carrot, Cedar, Chamomile, Cinnamon, Citron Lemon, Common Sage, Elecampane, Firs, Garlic, Inula, Juniper, Lemon, Mints, Nutmeg, Onion, Orange, Petitgrain (Combava), Pines, Rose Geranium, Rosemary, Savory, Tangerine, Tea Tree, Thyme, Vervain.

Cirrhosis: Also see *Liver*. Seek medical help. Birch, Boldo, Carrot, Elder, Juniper, Onion, Rosemary.

Cold Extremities: See *Circulation*.

Colds: See Bronchitis and Influenza. Angelica, Basil, Cinnamon, Dill, Eucalyptus, Hyssop, Juniper, Lavandin, Lavender, Lemon, Mints, Niaouli, Nutmeg, Rosemary, Sage, Thyme, Wild Thyme.

Rhinitis: Benzoin, Borneol, Eucalyptus, Lavender, Lemon, Marjoram, Mints, Niaouli, Onion, Peru Balsam, Pine, Thyme.

Hay fever (also see Asthma): Angelica, Eucalyptus, Fennel, Hyssop, Lavender, Marjoram, Melissa, Niaouli, St. John's Wort, Verbena.

Colic: Consult doctor.

Intestinal colic: Anise, Basil, Bergamot, Caraway, Chamomile, Common Sage, Cumin, Hyssop, Juniper, Marjoram, Melissa, Peppermint, Rosemary, Savory, Wild Thyme.

Gallstone: Anise, Boldo, Common Sage, Field Mint, Juniper, Nutmeg, Peppermint, Pine, Rosemary, Thyme, Visnaga.

Renal colic: Birch, Citron Lemon, Common Sage, Eucalyptus, Juniper, Peppermint, Visnaga.

Colitis (inflammation of the large intestine): See *Intestines*.

Condylome: (small skin growths which primarily grow around the anus or on the genital organs): Common Sage, Eucalyptus polybractea, Thyme (mild), Niaouli.

Congestion: (abnormal blood accumulation in part of the body):
Brain (stroke): Seek medical help. Hawthorne. *Phytotherapy*: Foot baths with Mustard.
Liver: Buchu. See *Liver*.
Lungs: Seek medical help. Eucalyptus, St. John's Wort.
Pelvis: Cypress, Thuja.
For external use: Lavender, Horseradish, Mustard, Rosemary.

Conjunctivitis, Blepharitis, Styes: Never put essential oils in the eyes!
External treatment with herb teas or hydrolates made of: Chamomile, Euphraisia, Mallow, Plantain.
Internal treatment with the following essential oils: Carrot, Clove, Fennel, Ginger, Chamomile, Lemon, Rosemary.

Constipation: Carrot, Chamomile, Coriander, Fennel, Juniper, Orange, Rose, Rosemary, Tarragon, Turpentine, Wild Thyme.

Contusions, Sprains, Dislocations: Chamomile, Cinnamon, Common Sage, Dill, Everlasting italicum, Hyssop, Lavender, Mace, Rosemary, Spike Lavender, Thyme.
Phytotherapy: Arnica Tincture.

Convalescence: Borneo Camphor, Cinnamon, Common Sage, Laurel, Lemon, Rosemary, Thyme, Wild Thyme.

Corns: Cade, Garlic, Myrtle, Spike Lavender, Thuja. *Phytotherapy*: fresh Celandine juice.

Coryza: See *Colds*.

Cough: Also see Bronchitis. China Anise, Cypress, Elecampane, Inula, Lavandin, Marjoram, Myrrh, Oriental Sweet Gum, Peru Balsam, Spike Lavender, Tarragon, Tolu Balsam.
Coughing fits, whooping-cough: Anise, Cypress, Eucalyptus, Origanum, Thyme, Valerian.

Cramps: Also see *Sedatives*.
Digestive system: Angelica, Anise, Basil, Cajeput, Caraway, Coriander.
Stomach: Cinnamon, Marjoram, Melissa, Peppermint.
Intestines: Anise, Bergamot, Cajeput, Caraway, Chamomile, Cinnamon, Cloves, Garlic, Juniper, Lavender, Lime, Myrtle, Nutmeg, Peppermint, Pine, Savory, St. John's Wort, Tea Tree, Turpentine, Wild Thyme.
Vascular: Cypress, Garlic.

Cramps in the Limbs: Anise, Chamomile, Common Sage, Gaultheria, Marjoram, Parsley, Valerian, Yellow Birch.
For external use: Borneo Camphor, Camphor, Lavandin, Marjoram, Peru Balsam, Rosemary.

Cuts, Fissures: Benzoin, Borneo Camphor, Carrot, Lemon, Onion, Peru Balsam, Sandalwood, Turpentine.

Dandruff: See *Hair Care*.

Deafness, Impaired Hearing: Caraway, Chamomile, Fennel, Garlic, Lemon, Onion, Savory. *For external use*: Dilute (5%) in olive or almond oil.

Demineralization (calcium deficiency): Celery, Common Sage, Lavender, Lemon, Rosemary.
Phytotherapy: Comfrey, Horsetail, Nettle. Also Magnesium Carbonate, Pollen.

Dermatitis: See *Skin Diseases*.

Diabetes: Consult doctor. Carrot, Chamomile, Citronella, Common Sage, Eucalyptus globulus, Fennel, Geranium, Juniper, Mints, Onion, Rosemary.

Diaper Rash: Carrot, Chamomile, Palmarosa (in 1-2% dilution in almond oil for external use).

Diarrhea (gastro-enteritis, dysentery): Angelica, Basil, Canadian Erigeron, Carrot, Chamomile, Cinnamon, Clove, Common Sage, Garlic, Gentian, Ginger, Juniper, Lavender, Lemon, Mace, Marjoram, Myrrh, Nutmeg, Orange, Peppermint, Rose Geranium, Sandalwood, Tansy, Wild Thyme.
Phytotherapy: Comfrey, Nettle.

Digestive Complaints: Anise, Basil, Bitter Orange, Caraway, Chamomile, Cinnamon, Clove, Common Sage, Coriander, Cumin, Dill, Fennel, Ginger, Hyssop, Juniper, Lavender, Lemon, Marjoram, Melissa, Mints, Nutmeg, Origanum, Rosemary, Savory, Sweet Flag, Tarragon, Thyme, Verbena, Wild Thyme.
Weak digestion: Bergamot, Caraway, Clary Sage, Origanum, Peppermint, Rosemary, Sweet Flag.
Painful digestion: Anise, Basil, Lavender, Peppermint, St. John's Wort, Sweet Flag.

Disinfection of Drinking Water: Lemon, Niaouli (after diluting 1:10 in 90% alcohol).

Disinfection of House and Room Air: Bupleurum, Cajeput, Eucalyptus, Fir, Grapefruit, Juniper, Lavender, Niaouli, Pine, Sage, Spruce.

Dislocations: See *Contusions*.

Diuretics: Anise, Birch, Caraway, Common Sage, Cypress, Dill, Fennel, Garlic, Juniper, Laurel, Lavender, Lemon, Onion, Orange, Origanum, Peppermint, Rosemary, Sassafras, Savory, Spike Lavender, Spiraea, Tarragon, Thyme, Turpentine, Wild Thyme.

Drunkenness: Stop drinking alcohol! Lemon, Parsley, Peppermint.
Phytotherapy: Cabbage, Horseradish, Leek, Onion.

Dysmenorrhea (painful periods): See *Periods*.

Dyspepsia (non-organic digestive disturbance): Also see *Flatulence* and *Digestion*.

Dysidrosis (itchy blisters between fingers and toes): Birch, Juniper, Parsley, Rosemary.
For external use: Cypress, Lavender, Pine, Sage.

Dystonia, Autonomic (disease of autonomic nervous system): Labdanum, Laurel, Lemongrass, Mountain Juniper, Peppermint, Petitgrain (Bitter Orange and Lemon), Sweet Marjoram, Tarragon, Wild Thyme.

Ear-Buzzing: Clarify possible causes (high blood pressure, arteriosclerosis, liver complaints, etc.). Melissa, Myrtle, Onion.

Eczema: *Dry*: Bergamot, Carrot, Cedar, Chamomile, Common Sage, Hyssop, Lavender, Rose Geranium, Rosemary.
Oozing: Cade (external use), Carrot, Chamomile, Common Sage, Hyssop, Juniper, Myrrh, Rosemary, Sassafras.

Edema: Consult doctor. Birch, Garlic, Juniper, Onion, Parsley, Turpentine.

Enteritis: See *Diarrhea*.

Enterocolitis: See *Intestine*.

Enterospasm: Angelica.

Epidemic (protection against infection): *For internal and external use and spraying:* Eucalyptus, Juniper, Lavender, Lemon, Niaouli, Pine, Tea Tree, Thyme.

Epilepsy: Consult doctor. Basil, Cajeput, Mandarin, Melissa, Parsley, Rosemary, Marjoram, Turpentine (in small doses), Thyme.

Exhaustion (nervous depression): Breathing and relaxation exercises, healthy eating habits, avoidance of stress. If necessary, remineralization (see Demineralization). Basil, Borneo Camphor, Carrot, Cat Mint, Chamomile, Common Sage, Incense, Lavender, Marjoram, Melissa, Nutmeg, Thyme, Wild Thyme.

Eyes: See *Conjunctivitis*. Never put essential oil in the eyes!

Facial Care: See *Skin*.

Fainting: *For external use*: Horseradish, Melissa, Mint, Mustard.

Fatigue: See *Asthenia* and *Anemia*.

Fermentation: See *Aerophagy* and *Intestinal Colic*.

Fever: Consult doctor if it lasts for more than one day or if it is very high. Angelica, Bergamot, Borneo Camphor, Cajeput, Chamomile, Cinnamon, Clove, Cypress, Eucalyptus, Garlic, Ginger, Lemon, Niaouli, Rosemary, Sage, Thyme, Wild Thyme, Ylang-Ylang.

Fibroma (benign fibrous tumor): Consult doctor. Common Sage, Cypress, Origanum. *Phytotherapy*: Comfrey, Horsetail, Milfoil, Nettle.

Flatulence: See *Aerophagy*.

Fleas: See *Parasites*, *Skin* and *Insect Bites*.

Frigidity: See *Impotence*

Frostbite: Borneo Camphor, Cedar, Celery, Chamomile, Lavender, Lemon, Niaouli, Onion, Peru Balsam, Rose Geranium, Spike Lavender. (Cold footbaths, twice daily.)

Gallbladder: Also see under *Liver* and *Gallstones*. Achillea Ligustica, Anise, Basil, Boldo, Calamint, Caraway, Carrot, Chamomile, Combava, Dill, Elecampana, Fennel, Hyssop, Juniper, Lavender, Lemon, Lovage, Mandarin, Melissa, Mugwort, Nutmeg, Onion, Peppermint, Rosemary, Sage, Savory, Spike Lavender, Thyme, Turmeric, Verbena, Wild Thyme.

Gallstones: Birch, Boldo, Carrot, Cat Mint, Fennel, Juniper, Lemon, Nutmeg, Onion, Pine, Rosemary, Turpentine.

Gas: See *Aerophagy*.

Glossitis (inflammation of the tongue): Also see *Gums*. Common Sage, Lemon, Juniper, Peppermint, Rose, Rose Geranium.

Goiter: Consult doctor. Garlic, Onion, Origanum Marjorana. For external use: Lavender, Rosemary.

Gout: Also see *Rheumatism*. Meatless diet. Avoid tomatoes, spinach, and stimulants. Basil, Birch, Cajeput, Canadian Erigeron, Chamomile, Elecampane, Garlic, Gentian, Juniper, Lemon, Pine, Rosemary, Thyme.
For external use: Pine, Sassafras, Turpentine.

Growth Disturbances: Carrot, Lemon, Onion, Parsley. *Phytotherapy*: Comfrey, Horsetail, Nettle.

Gums, Bleeding: See *Gums, Inflammation of*.

Gums, Inflammation of: Ceylon Cinnamon (bark), Fennel, Lemon, Origanum, Rose Geranium, Sage, Tea Tree.

Heat Blisters: *For external use:* Benzoin, Bergamot, Eucalyptus, Lavandin, Lavender, Lemon, Rose Geranium.

Hemorrhage: See *Bleeding*.

Hemorrhoids: Also see *Bleeding*. Non-irritating diet. Lavender to be used externally.

Hair Care:
Oily hair: Cedar, Lavender, Lemon, Pine
Dry hair: Melissa, Rose Geranium, Rosemary, Wild Thyme, Ylang-ylang.
Normal hair: Common Sage, Thyme.
Dandruff: Lavender and Cade (0.5%).

Hair Loss (circular bald spots, alopecia areata): Also see Baldness. Garden Sage, Clary Sage.

Harvest Mites (trombidioisis): See *Insect Bites*.

Hay Fever: See *Colds*.

Headaches: See *Migraine*.

Heart (disorders of cardiac rhythm): See *Palpitations*.

Heartburn: Non-irritating diet. Chamomile, Common Sage, Inula, Juniper, Lemon, Peppermint, St. John's Wort, Sweet Flag.
Phytotherapy: Comfrey, Gentian Root, Milfoil.

Hemiplegia (paralysis of one side of the body): Support of medical treatment: Cypress, Sweet Clover, Valerian.

Hepatitis, Viral: Basil, Bay, Clove, Laurel, Myrrh, Niaouli, Ravensara, Rosemary, Tea Tree.

Herpes (viral skin disease with outbreaks of blisters on the face and genitals):
Lemon, Rose Geranium, Savory.
For external treatment: Hyssop, Juniper, Lavender, Savory.

Hiccups: Anise, Calamint, Caraway, Coriander, Cumin, Dill, Fennel, Mandarin, Marjoram, Melissa, Origanum, Tarragon.

Hoarseness: Chinese Anise, Cypress, Lemon, Pennyroyal, Rose, Sweet Flag, Thyme.

Hot Flashes: Common Sage, Cypress, Valerian.
Also see *Menopause*.

Hyperchloremia (excess chloride in blood): Birch, Elder, Fennel, Inula, Onion, Parsley.

I
mpetigo (pustular skin disease with crust formation):
See *Skin Disease*.

Impotency: Anise, Borneo Camphor, Canaga, Chinese Anise, Cinnamon, Clove, Ginger, Juniper, Nutmeg, Onion, Peppermint, Pine, Rose, Rosemary, Rosewood, Sandalwood, Savory, Ylang-Ylang.

Indigestion: See *Digestive Complaints*.

Infectious Diseases: Almost all of the essential oils are antiseptic and bactericidal.

The following are particularly effective for:

Infections of the respiratory tract: Cajeput, Clove, Common Sage, Cypress, Eucalyptus, Hyssop, Lavender, Origanum, Niaouli, Pine, Sassafras, Thyme, Wild Lemon Thyme.

Intestinal infections: Basil, Bergamot, Chamomile, Cinnamon, Geranium, Lavender, Mace, Mints, Myrrh, Niaouli, Origanum, Rosemary, Thyme, Verbena, Visnaga, Wild Lemon Thyme.

Infections of the uro-genital region: Cajeput, Common Sage, Eucalyptus, Fennel, Juniper, Lavender, Lemon, Niaouli, Origanum, Pine, Rose Geranium, Sandalwood, Sassafras, Thyme, Wild Lemon Thyme.

Influenza: Cajeput, Chamomile, Cinnamon, Clove, Cypress, Eucalyptus, Garlic, Hyssop, Lavender, Lemon, Niaouli, Peru Balsam (external use), Pine, Ravensara, Rosemary, Sage, Spruce, Thyme.

Injuries (wounds, cuts): Benzoin, Bergamot, Cajeput, Canada Balsam, Chamomile, Copaiva, Cypress, Dill, Elemi, Eucalyptus, Everlasting italicum, Galbanum, Hyssop, Incense, Juniper, Lavandin, Lavender, Lemon, Nana Mint, Niaouli, Rose Geranium, Rose, Sage, Spike Lavender, Sweet Oriental Gum, Sweet Flag, Sweet Thyme, Tansy, Tea Tree, Thuja, Thyme.

Insect Bites and Stings: Bergamot, Chamomile, Common Sage, Cypress, Lavandin, Lavender, Lemon, Niaouli, Nutmeg, Onion, Palmarosa, Patchouli, Peppermint, Rose Geranium, Sassafras, Spike Lavender.

Insomnia:

Caused by nervousness: Angelica, Anise, Basil, Marjoram, Melissa, Petitgrain (Combava), Tangerine, Valerian, Vervain.

Caused by digestive disorders: Angelica, Anise, Basil, Chamomile, Lavender, Mandarin, Marjoram, Melissa, Orange, Verbena.

Caused by the liver (waking up around 3 am): Boldo, Fennel, Juniper.

Caused by heart and circulatory complaints or respiratory ailments: Anise, Hawthorne, Lavender, Thyme, Valerian.

Intestinal Parasites: See *Parasites*.

Intestines: (colitis, enterocolitis, inflammations, infections): Anise, Basil, Bay, Bergamot, Cajeput, Cubeb, Chamomile, Cinnamon, Combava, Juniper, Lavandins, Lavender, Leek, Mace, Mustard, Myrrh, Niaouli, Nutmeg, Patchouli, Peppermint, Rose Geranium, Rosemary, Savory, Thyme, Verbena, Wild Thyme, Ylang-ylang.

Irritability, Nervous: Achillea Ligustica, Agastache, Angelica, Anise, Basil, Chamomile, Citron Lemon, Cypress, Juniper, Lavender, Lemon, Marjoram, Orange, Spike Lavender, Tangerine.

Itching: Chamomile, Cedar, Clary Sage, Peppermint (for external use in 3% dilution).

For external genitals: Bergamot, Chamomile, Mild Thyme, Rose Geranium (for external use in 3% dilution).

Anus: Lavender, Rose Geranium, Rosemary (for external use).

Jaundice: See *Liver*

Kidney and Bladder Disorders (infections): Also see *Bladder Infection* and *Nephritis*. Angelica, Birch, Buchu, Cajeput, Canada Balsam, Chamomile, Clove, Common Sage, Copaiba balsam, Cubeb, Fennel, Guajac, Gurjun, Juniper, Lavender, Lemon, Niaouli, Nutmeg, Onion, Peppermint, Peru Balsam, Pine, Rosemary, Sandalwood, Sassafras, Turpentine, Thyme, Tolu Balsam, Wild Thyme.

Kidney Stones: Birch, Common Sage, Elecampana, Eucalyptus, Fennel, Garlic, Hyssop, Juniper, Lemon, Rose Geranium, Wild Thyme.

Lactation: See *Breast-Feeding*.

Laryngitis (inflammation of the larynx): Cajeput, Carrot, Common Sage, Lavender, Parsley, Pine, Rose Geranium, Wild Thyme.

Legs, Swollen: Clarify cause. Common Sage, Elder, Parsley, Rose Geranium.

Trace elements: Manganese and Cobalt.

Leucorrhea: Non-irritating diet. Benzoin, Cajeput, Chamomile, Cinnamon, Common Sage, Copaiba balsam, Cubeb, Eucalyptus, Incense, Juniper, Lavender, Lemon, Mild Thyme. Niaouli, Parsley, Peppermint, Rosemary, Sandalwood, Sassafras.

Lice: See *Parasites*, *Skin*.

Liver (disorders, diseases, jaundice): Achillea Lingustica, Agastache, Anise, Basil, Birch, Boldo, Carrot, Celery, Chamomile, Combava, Dill, Elecampane, Fennel, Gentian, Juniper, Lemon, Lovage, Mugwort, Pennyroyal, Peppermint, Petitgrain (Bitter Orange), Ravensara, Rosemary, Sage, Wintergreen, Wormwood, Yellow Birch.

Phytotherapy: Artichoke, Horseradish Juice, Dandelion Tincture.

Lumbago: Cajeput, Chamomile, Eucalyptus, Ginger, Lavender, Marjoram, Sassafras, Turpentine.

Lung Disorders: Cajeput, Clove, Common Sage, Cypress, Eucalyptus,

Fennel, Hyssop, Lavender, Citron, Lemon, Niaouli, Petitgrain (Bitter Orange), Pine, Sandalwood, Tea Tree, Turpentine.

Lungs, Emphysema of the: See *Pulmonary Emphysema.*

Lungs, Tuberculosis of the: See *Pulmonary Tuberculosis.*

Lupus (tubercular skin disease): Consult doctor. Clove, Rosemary, Savory, Thyme.

For external use: Benzoin, Incense, Myrrh, Peru Balsam.

Lymph Nodes, Enlarged: Birch, Carrot, Common Sage, Goldenrod, Myrtle, Rosemary, Pine.

Malaria: Angelica, Bergamot, Birch, Cinnamon, Cloves, Cypress, Eucalyptus globulus, Gentian, Laurel, Lemon, Lemongrass, Niaouli, Nutmeg, Origanum, Parsley, Savory, True Chamomile, Valerian, Verbena.

Measles, German Measles, Scarlet Fever, Smallpox: Angelica, Bergamot, Borneo Camphor, Cajeput, Camphor, Chamomile, Cinnamon, Cypress, Eucalyptus, Garlic, Labdanum, Lavender, Niaouli, Nutmeg, Peppermint, Ravensara, Spike Lavender, Thyme.

Memory, Poor: Basil, Clove, Common Sage, Coriander, Lemon, Onion, Parsley, Rosemary, Savory.

Meningitis: (inflammation caused by microbes or viruses): Consult doctor immediately! Cinnamon, Common Sage, Lemon, Thyme.

Menopause Disorders: Anise, Chamomile, Chinese Anise, Clary Sage, Common Sage, Cypress, Garlic, Hawthorne, Juniper, Lavender, Mandarin, Neroli, Orange, Parsley, Peppermint, Rosemary, Valerian.

Menstruation: See *Periods.*

Metritis (inflammation of the uterus): Also see *Leucorrhea.* Eucalyptus radiata, Fennel, Lemon, Origanum, Savory.

Migraines: Clarify cause (liver disorder, digestive disturbance, constipation, high blood pressure, backache).

Also see *Sedatives* and *Insomnia.* Anise, Basil, Chamomile, Eucalyptus, Lavender, Lemon, Marjoram, Melissa, Orange, Peppermint, Rosemary.

Milk Crust: Chamomile, Lavandin, Lavender.

Mosquito Repellent: Citronella, Clove, Eucalyptus, Lemongrass, Pennyroyal, Peppermint, Rose Geranium.

Moth Repellent: Clove, Lavandin, Lavender, Lemon, Vetiver.

Multiple Sclerosis: Bush Rosemary, Hyssop, Labdanum, Myrtle, Verbena.

Mumps: Consult doctor. Danger of genital, pancreatic, and meningeal complications. Chamomile, Cypress, Eucalyptus, Niaouli, Origanum, Sage, Spike Lavender.

Muscle Soreness: Chamomile, Juniper, Mace, Melissa, Mild Thyme, Peppermint, Rosemary.

For external use: Cinnamon, Pepper, Rosemary, Wild Thyme.

Muscular Rheumatism: Angelica, Borneo Camphor, Chamomile, Cinnamon, Common Sage, Cypress, Garlic, Lavandin, Lavender, Origanum, Pine, Rosemary, Rosemary, Tansy (annual), Thyme.

Mycosis: (fungal infection): Treat liver and intestinal flora. Carrot, Common Sage, Laurel, Lavandin, Lavender, Lovage, Mandarin, Mustard, Myrrh, Nana Mint, Niaouli, Patchouli, Rosewood, Savory, Tangerine, Tansy, Tea Tree, Thymes, Wood Mint.

Phytotherapy: Black Currant, Chervil, Marshmallow.

Nails, Brittle: Also see *Demineralization*. Lemon, Ylang-Ylang.

Nausea: Also see *Vomiting*. Clarify cause. Non-irritating diet. Angelica, Marjoram, Peppermint, Rosemary, St. John's Wort, Valerian.

Nephritis (inflammation of the kidneys): Angelica, Birch, Cajeput, Canadian Erigeron, Carrot, Chamomile, Eucalyptus, Fennel, Juniper, Lavender, Lemon, Niaouli, Peppermint, Rosemary, Thyme, Wild Thyme.

Nerves, Weak (neurasthenia): See *Anxiety*, *Asthenia*, and *Sedatives*.

Nervous System (to restore equilibrium): Cypress, Gentian, Marjoram, Rosemary, Spike Lavender.

Nervousness: See *Irritability* and *Sedatives*.

Nettle Rash: Clarify causes and treat.

Also see *Liver*, *Diuretics*, and *Blood Purification*. Antihistamines. Non-irritating diet. Benzoin, Bergamot, Common Sage, Juniper, Lavender, Myrrh, Palmarosa, Pine, Rose, Spike Lavender.

Neuralgia:

Dental: Cajeput, Clove, Juniper, Nutmeg, Peppermint.

Facial: Chamomile, Geranium, Peppermint (avoid eye contact!).

Sciatica, lumbago, intercostalneuralgia: Anise, Borneo Camphor, Chamomile, Eucalyptus, Ginger, Juniper, Lavandin, Lavender, Marjoram, Nutmeg, Pine, Rosemary, Sassafras, Spike Lavender, Turpentine, Vitiver, Wild Thyme.

Neurasthenia: See *Asthenia*.

Neuritis (inflammation of the nerves): Consult doctor. Achillea Ligustica, Cloves, Common Sage, Corkwood, Goldenrod, Laurel, Melissa, Mountain Juniper, Origanum, Peppermint, Rosemary, Spike Lavender, Tansy (annual), Tarragon, Thyme, Verbena.

Neurosis (nervous disorder): Basil (Eugenol), Sweet Marjoram.

Night Sweat: See *Sweating*.

Nosebleeds: Cypress, Turpentine, Wild Thyme.

Obesity: See *Weight-Reduction Diet* and *Diuretic*.

Oppression, Feeling of: See *Anxiety*.

Orchitis: (inflammation of the testicles) Consult doctor. Chamomile, Lemon, Origanum, Savory, St. John's Wort.

Otitis: (inflammation of the ear or middle ear): Consult doctor.
For internal use: Chamomile, Cinnamon, Eucalyptus radiata, Garlic, Lavender, Mild Thyme, Niaouli, Onion.
For external use: Eucalyptus radiata, Lavender (slightly diluted in plant oil).

Ovarian Insufficiency: Combava.

Overexertion (physical and mental): Also see *Asthenia*. Angelica, Anise, Basil, Coriander, Hyssop, Mace, Marjoram, Melissa, Neroli, Nutmeg, Orange, Parsley, Peppermint, Rosemary, Savory, Thyme.

Overweight: See *Weight-Loss Diet* and *Diuretics*.

Oxyuris: See *Parasites, Intestinal*.

Ozena (disorder of nasal mucous membrane accompanied by scabs and loss of sense of smell): Blood purifiers. Clary Sage, Common Sage, Eucalyptus radiata, Garlic, Juniper, Parsley.

Panaritium (circulation): Also see *Abscess*. Carrot, Onion, Roman Chamomile.

Polyarthritis, Rheumatic: Basil, Bay, Cajeput leucadendron, Clove, Common Sage, Eucalyptus, Gaultheria, Labdanum, Niaouli, Savory, Wintergreen.

Pyelitis: Everlasting gymnocephalum, Pine, St. John's Wort, Thyme, Turpentine.

Palpitations: Anise, Angelica, Canaga, Caraway, Hawthorne, Jatamansi, Large-Leafed Basil, Lavender, Neroli, Orange, Peppermint, Rosemary, Spike Lavender, Tangerine, Valerian, Ylang-Ylang.

Papilloma: See *Warts*.

Paralysis: Basil, Chamomile, Common Sage, Laurel, Marjoram, Melissa, Nutmeg, Rosemary, Thyme, Wood Mint.
Resulting symptoms: Chamomile, Juniper, Lavender, Rosemary.
Parkinson's Disease: Rosemary, Valerian; Arnica Tincture.

Parasites, Intestinal: Anise, Bergamot, Cajeput, Caraway, Cardamom,

Chamomile, Cinnamon, Clove, Common Tansy, Dill, Eucalyptus, Fennel, Garlic, Gentian, Goosefoot, Hyssop, Lavender, Lemon, Mace, Mugwort, Mustard, Myrrh, Neroli, Niaouli, Nutmeg, Onion, Pennyroyal, Peppermint, Santolina, Savory, Strong Thyme, Tagetes, Tansy, Tarragon, Thuja, Turpentine, Wild Thyme.

Eelworm: Goosefoot.

Hookworm: Goosefoot, Thyme.

Ascarids: Chamomile, Eucalyptus, Garlic, Goosefoot, Mugwort, Santolina, Thyme.

Oxyuris: Chamomile, Eucalyptus, Garlic, Goosefoot, Lemon, Mugwort, Thyme.

Tapeworms: Garlic, Thyme, Turpentine. *Phytotherapy*: Pumpkin seeds.

Whipworm: Thyme, True Chamomile. *Phytotherapy*: Pyrethrum, Tansy.

Parasites, Skin (lice, mites): Cade, Canada Balsam, Chamomile, Cinnamon, Clove, Common Tansy, Eucalyptus, Laurel, Lavender, Lemon, Lemongrass, Mustard, Niaouli, Nutmeg, Oriental Sweet Gum, Origanum, Pennyroyal, Peppermint, Peru Balsam, Rose Geranium, Rosemary, Spike Lavender, Sweet Lime, Thyme, Turpentine, Wild Thyme.

Pericarditis (inflammation of pericardium, membranous sac enclosing the heart):

Consult doctor. Birch, Goldenrod, Juniper, Onion.

Pediculosis: See *Parasites, Skin*.

Periods:

Missed: Chamomile, Common Sage, Common Tansy, Cypress, Elecampane, Mints, Mugwort, Origanum, Tagetes, Thyme.

Too light: Anise, Basil, Caraway, Carrot, Common Sage, Cumin, Fennel, Lavender, Lovage, Melissa, Mints, Mugwort, Nutmeg, Parsley, Rosemary, Santolina, Thyme, Wild Thyme-

Too heavy: Consult doctor. Cinnamon, Cypress, Juniper, Labdanum, Rose Geranium, Turpentine. *Phytotherapy*: Lady's Mantle, Milfoil Tincture.

Painful: Angelica, Anise, Cajeput, Chamomile, Common Sage, Cumin, Cypress, Elecampane, Juniper, Lovage, Mints, Mugwort, Parsley, Rosemary, Tarragon, Wild Thyme.

To regulate: Chamomile, Mints, Mugwort, Parsley. *Phytotherapy*: Marigold, Milfoil Tincture.

Pharyngitis (inflammation of pharyngeal mucosa): Cajeput, Ceylon Cinnamon, Creeping Hyssop, Eucalyptus globulus, Field Mint, Lavender, Niaouli, Palmarosa, Pine, Ravensara, Tea Trees.

Phlebitis (inflammation of vein walls): Consult doctor. Anise, Cypress, Everlasting Italicum, Lemon, Mastic Tree, Virginia Juniper.

Phlegmons (infection of cell tissue): Consult doctor. See *Abscess*.

Plethora (excess blood and fluid in the body): Consult doctor. Sudatory treatment. Birch, Elder, Horseradish, Hyssop, Juniper, Mustard, Onion.

Pneumonia: Consult doctor. Sudorific treatment. Borneo Camphor, Eucalyptus globulus, Horseradish, Lavender, Lemon, Mustard, Mustard, Niaouli, Pines, Tolu Balsam.

Polyps: Basil, Thuja.

Prostate Hypertrophy: Consult doctor. Agastache, Birch, Buchu, Cypress, Green Myrtle, Long-Leafed Basil, Onion, Peppermint, Spiraea, Thuja, Tolu Balsam.

Phytotherapy: Bearbeny, Heather, Horsetail.

For infections: Birch, Buchu, Common Pine, Juniper, Myrtle.

Psoriasis (skin disease with red scaly patches): Benzoin, Bergamot, Birch, Cajeput, Jatamansi, Lavender, Lovage, Wood Mint.

Psychoasthenia: Also see *Anxiety* and *Sedatives*. Anise, Basil, Lavender, Marjoram, Sage, Thyme, Valerian, Wild Thyme.

Pulmonary Emphysema: Cypress, Eucalyptus, Garlic, Hyssop, Lavender, Onion, Tansy (annual), Thyme.

Pulmonary Tuberculosis: Consult doctor. Benzoin, Borneo Camphor, Cajeput, Canada Balsam, Carrot, Clove, Common Sage, Cypress, Eucalyptus, Garlic, Gurjun Balsam, Horseradish, Juniper, Mustard, Myrtle, Neroli, Niaouli, Pepper, Peppermint, Peru Balsam, Pine, Rose, Thyme, Tolu Balsam, Turpentine.

Pyrosis: See *Heartburn*.

Rickets: Angelica, Basil, Carrot, Chamomile, Common Sage, Ginger, Horseradish, Juniper, Lavender, Lemongrass, Mild Thyme, Nutmeg, Onion, Parsley, Peppermint, Rosemary, Savory, Wild Thyme.

Rheumatism (arthritis, arthrosis): Achillea Liguistica, Angelica, Basil (Eugenol), Birch, Borneo Camphor, Cajeput, Camphor, Canadian Erigeron, Celery, Chamomile, Common Sage, Cypress, Eucalyptus, Fennel, Guajac, Galbanum, Garlic, Hyssop, Juniper, Laurel, Lavandin, Lavender, Lemon, Lovage, Mace, Mints, Niaouli, Nutmeg, Onion, Origanum, Pepper, Petitgrain (Combava), Pine, Rosemary, Sassafras, Savory, Tarragon, Thyme, Turpentine, Vetiver, Wild Thyme, Wintergreen.

Rhinitis: See *Colds*.

Rhinopharyngitis: See *Tonsillitis*.

Salpingitis (inflammation of Fallopian tubes): Chamomile, Eucalyptus, Lemon, Origanum, Sandalwood, Savory, St. John's Wort. *Phytotherapy*: Burdock, Lady's Mantle.

Scabies: Cinnamon, Clove, Garlic, Lavender, Lemon, Peppermint, Rosemary, Thyme, Turpentine.

Scabs: See *Milk Crust*.

Scarlet Fever: See *Measles*.

Sciatica: See *Neuralgia*.

Scrofula (disease of lymph nodes with tendency to chronic infections, often caused by eating habits): Also see *Lymph Nodes* and *Anemia*. Carrot, Cedar, Celery, Lavender, Onion, Pine, Horseradish, Common Sage, Thyme.

Scurvy: Carrot, Garlic, Ginger, Horseradish, Lemon, Onion, Orange, Parsley.

Seborrhea (excessive discharge from sebaceous glands): See *Hair Care*.

Sedatives: *The effect is often general; effects on specific organs are in parentheses.* Achillea Ligustica (relaxing), Angelica (nerves, digestion), Anise (nerves, digestion, heart and circulation, muscles), Basil, Bitter Orange (nervous system beneath diaphragm), Cat Mint, Citron Lemon (nerves), Common Sage (nerves, digestion, respiratory), Corkwood, Eucalyptus citriodora, Everlasting gymnocephalum, Fennel (nerves, digestion, insomnia), Giant Fir, Goldenrod (nerves), Hyssop officinalis, Jatamansi, Lavandin, Lavender (cerebro-spinal excitability, respiration, heart, insomnia), Lemon Tea Tree (digestion), Lemon Thyme, Mandarin (heart and circulation, insomnia, regulation of sympathetic nervous system), Marjoram (psychic, sympathetic nervous system, nerves, digestion, genital organs, insomnia), Melissa (excitability, nervous insomnia, migraines, spasms, vertigo, asthma), Mountain Juniper, Neroli (heart and circulation, palpitations, digestion, insomnia), Niaouli, Orange (nerves, digestion, insomnia), Petitgrain (Combava), Petitgrain (Mandarin), Ravensara, Roman Chamomile, Sandalwood (nerves and psyche), Sea Pine, Siberian Pine, Small-Leafed Sage, Spike Lavender (cerebrospinal overexcitability), Tangerine (sedative, relaxing), Tansy, Tea Tree, (balancing for sympathetic and parasympathetic nervous system), Thuja (urinary tract, prostate), Thyme (nerves, digestion, spasms), Verbena (nerves, digestion, vertigo), Ylang-Ylang (respiration, palpitations, overexcitability).

Shingles: Consult doctor. Benzoin, Carrot, Cloves, Common Sage, Cypress and Magnesium, Eucalyptus, Juniper, Lavender, Mints, Myrrh, Niaouli, Ravensara, Rose Geranium, Rosemary, Spike Lavender, Thuja, Thyme, Wintergreen.

Shock, Trauma, Accidents: Angelica, Carrot, Common Sage, Coriander, Everlasting Italicum, Juniper, St. John's Wort.
Phytotherapy: Arnica Tincture.

Sight, Poor:
For internal use: Carrot, Chamomile, Parsley, Rose, Rosemary.
Phytotherapy: Carrot, Blueberry.

Sinusitis: Non-toxic diet. Borneo Camphor, Calamint, Camphor, Chamomile, Eucalyptus, Iris, Juniper, Lavandin, Lavender, Lemon, Mints, Niaouli, Pines, Tagetes, Tansy, Thyme.

Skin and Facial Care: Benzoin, Bergamot, Carrot, Cedar, Chamomile, Clary Sage, Incense, Lavandin, Lavender, Lemon, Myrrh, Neroli, Orange, Palmarosa, Patchouli, Rose, Rose Geranium, Rosemary, Rosewood, Sandalwood, Spike Lavender, Vetiver, Ylang-Ylang.

Oily skin: Benzoin, Carrot, Chamomile, Common Sage, Lavender, Marjoram, Orange, Origanum, Patchouli, Wood Mint.

Dry skin: Benzoin, Carrot, Common Sage, Juniper, Lemon, Origanum, Palmarosa, Patchouli, Rosemary.

Impure skin (blackheads, acne): Cajeput, Clary Sage, Common Sage, Lavender, Palmarosa, Patchouli, Rose Geranium, Sandalwood, St. John's Wort.

Wrinkles: Carrot, Lavender, Lemon, Orange, Origanum, Palmarosa, Patchouli, Rose Geranium, Rose, Rosemary, Sandalwood.

Anti-wrinkle oils: 2 ml each of Carrot, Origanum, and Rosemary in wheatgerm, almond, and olive oil (30 ml of each). Or: 2 ml each of Lavender, Lemon, and Rose Geranium in wheatgerm, sesame, and sunflower oil (30 ml of each).

Skin Disease (dermatosis): Non-irritating diet, blood purifier, derivant. Angelica, Benzoin, Bergamot, Birch, Borneo Camphor, Cade, Camphor, Canada Balsam, Carrot, Cedar, Chamomile, Clary Sage, Clove, Common Sage, Cypress, Elemi, Eucalyptus, Garlic, Gurjun, Hyssop, Incense, Laurel, Lavandin, Lavender, Lemon, Mints, Mustard, Myrrh, Myrtle, Neroli, Niaouli, Nutmeg, Onion, Orange, Oriental Sweet Gum, Origanum, Palmarosa, Parsley, Patchouli, Peru Balsam, Rose, Rose Geranium, Rosemary, Sandalwood, Spike Lavender, Tansy, Tansy (annual), Thuja, Thyme, Tolu Balsam, Turpentine, Wild

Thyme, Ylang-Ylang.

Skin Proliferations: Basil, Hyssop, Thuja.

Phytotherapy: Icelandic Lichen, Oyster Shells, Sorrel Root.

Smoking, Discontinuing: Anise, Cinnamon, Clove, Common Sage, Lemon, Sassafras, Savory.

Inhalation: Mixture of Coriander, Eucalyptus camaldulensis, Fennel, Origanum, Rose Geranium, and Sassafras. Acupuncture and ear acupuncture.

Snake Bites: Consult doctor. Anti-venom serum. Lavender, Onion.

Spasmophilia: Cajeput, Cat Mint, Chamomile, Goldenrod, Jatamansi, Peppermint, Ravensara, Tarragon, Valerian.

Spleen Insufficiency: Peppermint, St. John's Wort, Verbena, Wood Mint.

Phytotherapy: Buckthorn Bark, Garden Sorrel, Milk Thistle.

Sprains: See ***Contusions***.

Sterility: Borneo Camphor, Common Sage, Coriander, Hyssop, Juniper, Nutmeg, Onion, Parsley, Peppermint, Rose, Rose Geranium, Savory.

Stimulants:

For the leucocytosis (production of white blood corpuscles): Lemon, Thyme.

For the brain: Basil, Clove, Nutmeg, Onion, Rosemary, Savory, Thyme.

For blood circulation: Caraway, Cinnamon, Common Sage, Garlic, Nutmeg, Thyme.

For digestion: Anise, Caraway, Chamomile, Fennel, Garlic, Juniper, Verbena.

For the respiratory tract: Anise, Chamomile, Cinnamon, Garlic, Pine, Ravensara.

For the nervous system: Basil, Fennel, Juniper, Lemon, Onion, Peppermint, Rosemary, Sage, Thyme.

General: Anise, Chamomile, Clove, Common Sage, Coriander, Eucalyptus, Fennel, Garlic, Geranium, Juniper, Lavender, Lemon, Nutmeg, Onion, Peppermint, Rosemary, Sassafras, Savory, Tarragon, Thyme.

Stomach Pain (gastritis): Also see ***Aerophagy***, ***Heartburn***, and ***Digestive Complaints***. Angelica, Anise, Anise-Ravensara, Caraway, Cardamom, Cinnamon, Fennel, Lemon, Mandarin, Rosemary, Savory, St. John's Wort, Tangerine, Tarragon.

Stomatitis (inflammation of mucous membrane of the mouth): Also see ***Gums***. Juniper, Laurel, Lemon, Rose Geranium, Sage, Stoechas Lavender, Tansy, Tea Tree.

Sunburn: The same essential oils as for Burns, but diluted in oil (25% of essential oil in almond, olive, or sesame oil.)

Sweating, Excessive: Eucalyptus, Hyssop, Juniper, Lemon, Marjoram, Niaouli, Nutmeg, Onion, Parsley, Peppermint, Sage, Savory, Thuja, Thyme, Wild Thyme.

Syphilis, Gonorrhea: Consult doctor. Bergamot, Cajeput, Canada Balsam, Cubeb, Guajak, Garlic, Juniper, Lemon, Niaouli, Parsley, Pepper, Peru Balsam, Pine, Sandalwood, Sassafras, Sweet Oriental Gum, Tolu Balsam, Turpentine.

Tapeworm: See *Parasites, Intestinal.*

Testicles, Insufficiency of: Combava.

Tetany (painful muscular spasms): Consult doctor. Mild Thyme and Origanum and Parsley. Calcium and Magnesium.

Thinness, Weight Loss: Consult doctor. *Appetite-stimulating and strengthening essential oils*: Carrot, Common Sage, Ginger, Onion, Rosemary.
Phytotherapy: Fenugreek seeds, Vitamins from the B group.

Ticks: Lavender, Marjoram (drop directly onto tick).

Tinea: See *Skin Diseases.* Benzoin, Birch, Carrot, Chamomile, Common Sage, Elder, Lemon, Peru Balsam, Rose Geranium, Tolu Balsam, Verbena.

Tonsillitis (infectious throat inflammation):
Basil (Eugenol), Chamomile, Clove, Common Sage, Eucalyptus, Green Myrtle, Inula, Laurel, Lavender, Lemon, Niaouli, Pepper, Rose, Tea Tree.
Streptococcal anina (white spots on tonsils): Chamomile, Lemon, Niaouli, Parsley, Ravensara.
Angina pectoris: Anise.
Vincent's Angina: Peppermint.

Tooth Care: Also see *Demineralization.* Chamomile, Clove, Lemon, Sage, Thyme.
Phytotherapy: Horsetail.

Torticollis (wryneck): Borneo Camphor, Cinnamon, Marjoram.
For external use: Camphor, Chamomile, Lavandin, Marjoram, Turpentine.

Tumors: See *Cancer.*

Typhoid Fever: Consult doctor. Borneo Camphor, Cinnamon, Garlic, Lavender, Lemon, Thyme.

Follow-up treatment: See ***Intestines***.

Ulcers: *Stomach and intestinal ulcers*: Relaxation, reduction of stress, breathing exercises, eat in a calm atmosphere.
Angelica, Anise, Carrot, Chamomile, Lemon, Sage.
Phytotherapy: Comfrey, Liquorice, Marigold, Nettle.
For external use: Carrot, Chamomile, Clary Sage, Common Sage, Garlic, Incense, Labdanum, Lavender, Mints, Myrrh, Onion, Rose, Rosemary, St. John's Wort, Thyme.
On the legs: Also see Wounds, Poorly healing. Carrot, Celery, Common Sage, Garlic, Incense, Juniper, Labdanum, Lantana, Myrrh, Oriental Sweet Gum, Pine, Rose Geranium, St. John's Wort, Wild Thyme.

Uremia (excess uric acid in the blood): Monitoring by doctor. Angelica, Birch, Carrot, Common Sage, Eucalyptus dives, Fennel, Juniper, Lavender, Marjoram, Mint, Onion, Pine, Rosemary, Sweet Flag, Thyme, Wild Thyme.
Phytotherapy: Artichoke, Dandelion.

Urethritis (inflammation of the ureter): Consult doctor. Bay, Buchu, Cajeput, Cedar, Eucalyptus, Fennel, Giant Fir, Gurgun Balsam, Mild Thyme, Myrrh, Myrtle, Niaouli, Palmarosa, Parsley, Patchouli, Peru Balsam, Sandalwood, Tansy, Tea Tree, Tolu Balsam, Turpentine, Wild Lemon Thyme.

Urine, Blood in (ecchymosis): See ***Contusions***.

Urine Excretion, Inadequate (oliguria): Consult doctor. Drink water and herb teas. Anise, Birch, Carrot, Common Sage, Fennel, Juniper, Lavender, Lovage, Mints, Onion, Spiraea, Thyme, Wild Thyme.

Uterus: *Inflammation*: Consult doctor. Canada Balsam, Chamomile, Clary Sage, Melissa, Parsley.
Phytotherapy: Lady's Mantle, Milfoil.
As stimulant: Clove, Incense, Melissa, Mugwort, Myrrh, Nutmeg, Pennyroyal.

Vaginitis: Canada Balsam, Ceylon Cinnamon, Chamomile, Clary Sage, Eucalyptus globulus, Palmarosa, Parsley, Peru Balsam, Rosewood, Sandalwood.

Varicose Veins: Agastache, Cajeput, Chamomile, Clary Sage, Cypress, Eucalyptus radiata, Garlic, Jatamansi, Juniper, Lavender, Lemon, Mastic Tree, Niaouli, Onion, Patchouli, Rose Geranium, Rosemary, Sandalwood, Tansy (annual), Thyme.
Phytotherapy: Milk Thistle, Witch Hazel, Indian Chestnut, Wild

Pansy, Red Vine.

Vertigo: Medical diagnosis. Angelica, Anise, Basil, Bitter Orange, Camphor, Caraway, Cardamom, Chamomile, Hawthorne, Lavender, Lemon, Mandarin, Marjoram, Melissa, Mugwort, Neroli, Orange, Peppermint, Rosemary, Sage, Sweet Lime, Thyme.

Voice, Loss of: See *Aphony* and *Hoarseness*.

Vomiting: Medical diagnosis. Common Sage, Dill, Lemon, Peppermint, Rosemary.

Due to pregnancy: Melissa, Nutmeg, Peppermint.

Nervous Vomiting: Angelica, Anise, Cajeput.

Warts: Cinnamon (bark), Garlic, Lemon, Onion, Thuja.

Phytotherapy: Celandine, Marigold.

Weakness, General Fatigue: See *Asthenia* and *Anemia*.

Weight-Loss Diet (cellulite, obesity): Study the endocrine terrain. Basil, Celery, Common Sage, Garlic, Grapefruit, Juniper, Lavender, Lemon, Onion, Orange, Origanum, Rosemary, Thyme.

For external use: Cedar, Cypress, Juniper, Origanum.

Whooping Cough: Anise, Basil, Chamomile, Cypress, Eucalyptus, Garlic, Lavender, Niaouli, Pine, Rosemary, Thyme, Wild Thyme.

Worms: See *Parasites, Intestinal*.

Wounds:

Poorly healing: Benzoin, Cajeput, Carrot, Clove, Common Sage, Garlic, Juniper, Lavender, Mild Thyme, Myrrh, Niaouli, Onion, Oriental Sweet Gum, Origanum, Rose, Rosemary, Savory, Spike Lavender, St. John's Wort.

Infected wounds: Anise, Benzoin, Bergamot, Cajeput, Canada Balsam, Chamomile, Clove, Common Sage, Cypress, Eucalyptus, Garlic, Hyssop, Lavender, Lemon, Mild Thyme, Oriental Sweet Gum, Palmarosa, Patchouli, Peru Balsam, Rose, Rose Geranium, Rosemary, Savory, Spike Lavender, Tolu Balsam, Wild Thyme.

Wrinkles: Carrot, Clary Sage, Lemon, Neroli, Orange, Palmarosa, Patchouli, Rose, Rosewood.

Y ellow Fever: Peppermint.

Remedies for Supporting Terrain Treatment

The following brief index lists essences which are suitable for a terrain cure. This index and the previous one should be consulted together. (See instructions at the beginning of the chapter.)

Albuminuria: See *Albumin*.

Anti-Cholesterol: See *Cholesterol*.

Anti-Diabetic (lowers blood sugar levels): Birch, Carrot, Celery, Chamomile, Common Pine, Common Sage, Eucalyptus, Everlasting gymnocephalum, Fennel, Garlic, Geranium, Hyssop, Juniper, Mild Thyme, Onion, Peppermint, Rosemary.

Anti-Rheumatic: See *Rheumatism* in therapeutic index.

Blood Pressure, High and Low: See therapeutic index.

Bodily Fluids: *Drainage*: Eucalyptus radiata, derivants, diuretics. *Phytotherapy*: Burdock Root.

Cerebro-Spinal Excitability: *Sedation*: Lavender, Spike Lavender.

Cholagogue (stimulates the liver function and increases the flow of bile): Birch, Boldo, Boxwood, Carrot, Chamomile, Juniper, Lavender, Pennyroyal, Rosemary.

Suprarenal Cortex: *Stimulation*: Basil, Borneo Camphor, Celery, Cinnamon, Clary Sage, Common Pine, Common Sage, Niaouli, Rose Geranium, Rosemary, Savory, Spruce, Thyme.
Reduction: Angelica, Verbena, Ylang-Ylang.

Diuretics:
General: Birch, Buchu, Canadian Erigeron, Caraway, Celery, Common Sage, Cumin, Cypress, Dill, Elder, Fennel, Garlic, Goldenrod, Hyssop, Juniper, Laurel, Lavender, Leek, Lemon, Lovage, Mastic Tree, Mint, Onion, Orange, Origanum, Parsley, Peru Balsam, Radish, Rosemary, Sassafras, Savory, Spike Lavender, Tarragon, Thuja, Thyme, Turpentine, Wild Thyme.
Urinary antiseptic: Buchu, Juniper, Melissa, Sandalwood, Sweet Clover, Thuja.
Promotes elimination of urea: Birch, Celery, Elecampane, Fennel, Inula, Linden Sapwood, Onion.
Promotes elimination of cholesterol: Boldo
Promotes elimination of chlorides: Birch, Elder, Elecampane, Fennel, Onion, Parsley.
Promotes elimination of uric acid: Birch.

Estrogen: Female hormone which triggers menstruation.

Febrifuge (essential oils which reduce fever): Angelica, Birch, Boxwood, Chamomile, Common Sage, Eucalyptus, Garlic, Ginger, Juniper, Laurel, Lemon, Niaouli, Orange, Palmarosa, Patchouli, St. John's Wort, Valerian, Verbena.

Gallbladder: *Stimulation*: Boldo, Mints, Rosemary.

Glandular System: *Stimulation*: Garlic, Onion.

Heart: *Stimulation*: Anise, Borneo Camphor, Caraway, Cinnamon, Garlic, Hawthorne, Inula, Lavender, Lemon, Rosemary.

Regulation of heart rhythm: See Palpitations in therapeutic index.

Hypothalamus: *Regeneration*: Bergamot.

Immune System: Ceylon Cinnamon, Eucalyptus Radiata, Incense, Labdanum, Niaouli, Origanum compactum, Ravensara, Savory, Tea Tree, Thyme.

Kidneys: *Stimulation*: Celery Seed, Grapefruit, Juniper, Onion, Opoponax, Peppermint, Thyme.

Regulation: Eucalyptus Dives.

Liver and Hepatic Functions: See *Liver* in therapeutic index.

Medulla Oblongata: *Stimulation*: Clary, Sage, Hyssop, Mild Thyme.

Menopause: See therapeutic index.

Menstruation: *To trigger or increase*: Angelica, Anise, Basil, Caraway, Chamomile, Cinnamon, Cumin, Fennel, Hyssop, Juniper, Lantana, Laurel, Lavender, Lovage, Marjoram, Mint, Mugwort, Origanum, Parsley, Ravensara, Rosemary, Sage, Tarragon, Thyme, Vetiver, Wild Thyme, Wormwood.

Nervous System

Sympathetic:

Stimulation: Basil, Common Sage, Lemon, Linden, Pine, Savory.

Sedation: Angelica, Hawthorne, Lavender, Mandarin, Marjoram, Orange, Spike Lavender, Sweet Clover, Ylang-Ylang.

Parasympathetic (Vagus):

Stimulation: Clove, Marjoram, Oregano, Rosemary, Verbena.

Sedation: Cajeput, Cypress, Hyssop, Tarragon, Wild Thyme.

Regulating for Sympathetic/Parasympathetic:

Common Sage, Gentian, Lemongrass, Peppermint, Verbena.

Ovaries

Estrogen:

Stimulation: Angelica, Anise, Cajeput, Caraway, Chinese Anise, Clary Sage, Common Sage, Coriander, Cypress, Fennel, Inula, Ravensara.

Phytotherapy: Chervil, Hops, Marigold, Saffron.

Reduction: Cumin. *Phytotherapy*: (Agnus castus)

Progesterone:

Stimulation: *Phytotherapy*: Lady's Mantle.

Pancreas: *Stimulation*: Lemon, Everlasting gymnocephalum, Juniper, Lemon, Onion, Petitgrain (Lemon), Rosemary, Thyme.

Pituitary Gland:

Stimulation: Inula, Niaouli

Reduction: Stoneseed (lithospermum).

Prostate: Hypertrophy. See therapeutic index.

Reticulo-Endothelial Terrain: Niaouli.

Rheumatism: See **Rheumatism** in therapeutic index.

Spleen: *Stimulation*: Chamomile, Fennel, Onion, Pennyroyal, Peppermint, Rose, St. John's Wort, Thyme, Wood Mint.

Sudorific (sweating-producing): Angelica, Anise, Carrot, Chamomile, Common Sage, Cumin, Cypress, Elecampane, Gentian, Hyssop, Juniper, Laurel, Lavender, Marjoram, Melissa, Peppermint, Rosemary, Sassafras, Spiraea, Sweet Flag, Thyme.

Sweat, Regulation: Angelica, Chamomile, Common Sage, Gentian, Laurel.

Thyroid: *Stimulation*: Algae (Fucus, Laminaria), Myrtle.

Phytotherapy: Oats

Reduction: Calamint, Cumin, Fennel.

Regulation (obesity, goiter): Origanum, Sweet Marjoram.

Vasoconstrictors: Cypress, Lemon.

Vasodilators: Garlic, Gaultheria, Hawthorne, Rosemary.

Chapter IX

Reference Section

Definitions

Abortifacient: Drug or other agent capable of causing abortion.

Adenitis: Acute or chronic inflammation of the Lymph nodes (head, thigh, in the groin).

Adjuvant: Complementary therapeutic aid.

Allergy: Any harmful change of the humoral environment, caused by some substance or other (for example, medications or certain foods).

Alopecia: Baldness with various causes: infectious diseases such as seborrhoea, mange, scabs, syphilis, and others.

Amenorrhea: Absence or cessation of menstruation with various causes.

Analgesic/Anodyne: Relieves pain.

Anorexia: Loss or reduction of appetite.

Anosmia: Total or partial loss of sense of smell, often accompanied with loss of sense of taste.

Anthelmintic: Vermifuge.

Antibiotic: Substance with "anti-life" effect, opposing the growth of microbes.

Antihistamine: Anti-allergic substance which counteracts the harmful effects of histamine (amine found in animal tissue, which can cause inflammation).

Antiphlogistic: Reducing inflammation. (Use through baths, compresses, emollients leeches).

Antiseptic: Destroys microbes and/or prevents their growth.

Apoplexy: Abrupt loss of consciousness or ability to move, which may be followed by paralysis which can be more or less permanent.

Arteriosclerosis: Thickening and hardening of the artery walls.

Arteritis: Inflammatory or degenerative arterial injury.

Arthritis: Inflammation of joints.

Arthritism: Specific state of the organism with a disposition toward gout, rheumatism, migraine, asthma, calculi, obesity, and diabetes. Its origin is associated with a slow self-poisoning, particularly caused by food which is too heavy and rich.

Asthenia: General exhaustion.

Astringent: Agent which causes contraction of tissue. Facilitates the healing of wounds and scar formation. Also reduces the flow of secretions.

Atony: Reduction of tone (muscle tension) in a contractile organ (for example, stomach).

Autonomic: The autonomic nervous system is the nervous system of the organs and intestines. It safeguards and regulates the so-called autonomic functions: respiration, circulation, metabolism, and reproduction. It is connected to the central nervous system.

Bactericide: Destroys bacteria.

Bacteriostatic: Inhibits bacterial growth.

Balsamic: Fragrance containing balm which perfumes, disinfects, and soothes.

Blepharitis: Inflammation of the eyelids, particularly the margins.

Bulimia: Excessive hunger to the point of gluttony.

Carditonic: Strengthens the heart.

Carminative: Promotes expulsion of intestinal gas.

Cephalalgia: Headache.

Chemotypes: One plant variety may sometimes include different chemical families chemotypes which are a variation of the main component of the respective essential oil. For example, Common Thyme includes thymol- and linalol-based thymes).

Cholagogue: General promotion of bile elimination.

Cholekinetic: Facilitates drainage of the gallbladder.

Choleretic: Stimulates the flow of bile.

Chromatography: Analytical method which makes it possible to separate the components of an essential oil from each other in order to identify them and determine their dosage. Within this process, the essential oil is subject to the effects of two phases in either a liquid or gaseous medium. One of these phases is mobile and the other is immobile. In accordance with its affinity with each phase, the essential oil is moved with greater or lesser speed and extent by the mobile phase.

Cirrhosis: Term used for several diseases of the liver (for example, alcoholic cirrhosis, tubercular cirrhosis, malarial cirrhosis).

Colitis, Enterocolitis: Inflammation of the large intestine and small intestine.

Depurative: Agent which helps remove impurities and toxins from the blood.

Derivant: Causes a sudden increase in the flow of blood, relieving congestion in an afflicted organ.

190

Dextrogyre: The property of causing polarized light rays to rotate to the right.

Diuretic: Causing an increased flow of urine.

Dropsy: Disease in which watery fluid collects in the natural cavities of the body (such stomach, meninges, and spinal meniges).

Dyshidrosis: Itchy eruption of small blisters between the fingers and toes.

Dyspepsia: Digestive complaints, disturbances, or weakness.

Dystonia: Disturbance of normal muscular and vascular tone.

Dystrophy: Changes in the shape and function of tissue, an organ, or gland, caused by a nutritional disturbance.

Emetic: Causing vomiting.

Emmenagogue: Promotes or regulates the menstrual flow.

Emollient: Relaxes and softens inflamed tissue and soothes inflammations.

Enterocolitis: See *Colitis*.

Enzyme: Protein which acts as a catalyst for a specific biochemical reaction, making this reaction possible (for example, digestion).

Expectorant: Promotes ejection of superfluous substances in the respiratory tract.

Febrifuge: Agent which reduces fever.

Flatulence (meteorism): Excessive formation of gas in the intestine and stomach, accompanied by wind.

Galactagogue: Promotes the flow of breast-milk.

Hemostatic: Stops bleeding.

Hookworm: Small cylindrical worm which nests in large numbers in the mucous lining of the small intestine and causes ancylostomiasis (anemia due to small but constant hemorrhage).

Hydrolate: Aromatic water obtained by steam being guided through the plants during distillation and then recovered after condensation.

Hypertensive: Increases blood pressure.

Hypnotic, Hypnagogic: Induces sleep.

Hypotensive: Decreases blood pressure.

Icterus: Jaundice.

Ketones: Simple chemical substances contained in various essential oils. They have aromatic and expectorant properties, but are toxic if taken in large quantities (for example, carvone and thuyone).

Laxative: Mild purgative, promoting evacuation of the bowels.

Levogyre: The property of causing polarized light rays to rotate to the left.

Lithiasis: Formation of gravel or calculi in the body (for example, kidney stones, gallstones, salivary calculus).

Menopause: Change of life.

Meteorism: Bloated abdomen due to intestinal gas.

Nephritis: Inflammation of the kidneys.

Neuritis: Inflammation of the nerves.

Ocytoxic: Hormone which facilitates birth.

Oleoresin: Term for an oil, resin, or essential oil obtained from a tree whose resin is collected for distillation (for example, Canada Balsam and Copaiba Balsam).

Pathogenic: Morbid factor leading to occurrence of disease.

Pectoral: Beneficial for the respiratory tract.

Peptic: Promotes digestion.

Phenols: 1. Derivate of benzene, one of the most commonly used antiseptics in hospitals. 2. Phenols present in essential oils, which also have a very antiseptic effect. These are important components of certain plants such as varieties of thyme and origanum, rosemary, savory, clove.

Pyorrhea: Infection process with formation of pus.

Pyrosis: Heartburn.

Refractive Index: Measurement for change of direction of light when it enters a second medium with different density. In our case this means the change effecting the essential oil.

Resolutive: Anticongestive agent.

Reticulo-Endothelial System (RES): The reticulo-endothelial tissue contains a large cell, the hemocytoblast, which produces blood corpuscles.

RF (Rheumatic Fever): Acute muscle rheumatism; inflammatory joint disease caused by streptococcus infection which can consecutively also spread to the heart.

Rubefacient: Agent which regulates skin heat and stimulates skin to redness.

Sedative: Agent with a calming effect.

Spectrography: Several methods of identifying the chemical substances present in a fluid by studying the spectrum of their light absorption.

Still: Distilling apparatus which looks like a large pressure-cooker and consists of a vat in which plants are placed and pressed together before they are steamed to draw out the essential oil. The steam then cools and condenses in the cooling coil, which ends in the essence bottle. Here the essential oil is collected as it floats on top of the distilled floral water, called hydrolate.

Stimulant: Agent which increases the activity of a function or an organ.

Stomachic: Promotes digestion.

Sudorific: Induces sweating.

Synergy: Combination of various elements which all strengthen their mutual effect.

Terpenes or Terpenoids: Very common organic hydrocarbon compounds present in essential oils (for example, pinene, camphene, limonene).

Tinctures, Mother Tinctures, Alcoholates: Various forms of plant macerations in alcohol.

The tinctures: 20% of weight of dried plants in 60% alcohol.

Mother tinctures: Form the basis of homeopathy using fresh plants whose proportion corresponds to 10% of their dried weight in 60% alcohol.

Alcoholates: 20% of fresh plants in 95% alcohol.

Tonic: Strengthening agent for improvement of tone (quick stimulant).

Vago-Sympathetic: The vagus nerve which begins in the medulla oblongata and guides the nerve stimuli to the bronchial tubes, the heart, the digestive system, and the kidneys. It is part of the parasympathetic sub-system.

Vasoconstrictive: Agent which narrows the blood vessels.

Vasodilating: Agent which dilates the blood vessels.

Vermifuge: Agent which causes intestinal worms to be expelled.

Vermicide: Agent which kills intestinal worms.

The Difference Between Aromatherapy and Related Natural Therapies

Biological Medicine or Naturopathy

According to naturopathy, each individual is responsible for the state of his or her own organism. Diseases are therefore not accidents, but the consequence of a certain way of living and eating which produces self-poisoning as the bodily fluids (blood, lymph, mucous) become saturated with too many deposits and waste materials. These humoral strains (such as crystallizations) are the deeper cause for the majority of our diseases. As a result, many symptoms which are called diseases are forms of auto-immune defense and our body's efforts to eliminate toxic waste. The attempt to suppress symptoms and excretions only leads to the ostensible restoration of health. However, in reality it frequently leads to neglecting the problem and paving the way for relapses and chronic conditions.

This is why naturopathy concentrates on determining the various deeper causes of an illness, taking into account how they effect the entire individual along with his or her natural and social background. Its main form of therapy includes all of the natural factors: air, water, sunshine, movement, exercise, positive thinking, a change in lifestyle and eating habits. Their objective is to detoxify the bodily fluids. If the patient's condition is serious, naturopathy will also make use of other natural therapies: phytotherapy, aromatherapy, homeopathy, etc.. If the patient's state of health cannot be improved by using these therapies, it has recourse to allopathy.

Materialistic thinking ascribes blind activity to the human body, giving the practicing physician the right to intervene in its mechanisms should they become disorderly.
In contrast, naturopathy takes into consideration that life, the living being, possesses intelligence. Life knows what it does. It can keep the organism in a good condition and, when necessary, heal it. In keeping with this idea, P. V. Marchesseau writes: "The naturopath does not heal in this sense; he helps strengthen the vital force, and it is the body which heals itself when it is ill."

There are two kinds of naturopathic treatments related to eating:

- Fasting: (See bibliography)
- Non-toxic diets.

194

The following should be avoided: stimulants (tea, coffee, cocoa, nicotine, alcohol); "dead" foods like canned foods and chemically treated, industrially produced, and refined products (sugar, white flour, etc.); fatty, red meats and sausages.

Eat the following as often as possible: raw vegetables, fruit, germinated wholegrain cereals, nuts (hazelnuts, almonds); drink good spring water, especially one glass before you go to bed and when you get up (possibly with lemon juice), as well as depurative and cleansing herb teas.

Homeopathy

Two thousand years ago, Hippocrates formulated two ways for medicine to proceed: "A disease can be treated through its opposite (the principle on which allopathy developed), and a disease can be healed through similitude." Samuel Hahnemann established homeopathy based on the latter principle during the nineteenth century. He observed that a substance which causes symptoms to appear in a healthy patient is able to heal the same symptoms and the disease which occurs because of them. Homeopathy is based on the following three main principles:

- *The law of similitude*: any substance capable of causing certain symptoms to appear in a healthy person is also liable to cause similar symptoms to disappear in a sick person.
- *The law of infinitesimality*: the therapeutic effect of a homeopathic dose increases with dilution. Consequentially, infinitesimal doses of active substances will have a greater therapeutic effect than a large dose of the same substance.
- *The law of individualization*: each individual reacts differently (according to his or her constitution, temperament, past experiences, etc.) to any disease. For this reason, homeopathy does not treat an illness, but heals a sick person. This individual is a complete entity and must therefore be treated as such. Homeopathy is therefore a personalized system of medicine.

The basic substances of homeopathy are the mother tinctures. These are mainly extracted from plants, but also from minerals and animals. The tinctures are diluted and dynamized, producing remedies available in the form of drops or globules. These substances primarily work on the energetic level by stimulating the auto-immune defence mechanisms and stimulating the restoration of equilibrium.

In the practice, homeopaths can be divided into two different categories: those who work with complex remedies tend to use the symptoms as a starting point and prescribe several medications at the same time. The other group, which works with simple remedies, attempts to understand the patient's organic terrain or environment, the general state of health, by using a long questionnaire. These homeopaths prescribe one medicament at a time (Similimum), which is meant to restore the equilibrium of the patient's overall constitution. This approach is more representative of the methods of homeopathy's founders Hahnemann and Kent. However, since it is more difficult to practise, there are fewer therapists who work with it.

Phytotherapy

Phytotherapy is the mother of all systems of medicine, particularly biological medicine and naturopathy. With the intention of extracting the natural active ingredients of plants, chemistry branched off from phytotherapy during the nineteenth century and developed the capacity of producing completely synthesized medicaments. At present, 40% of allopathic drugs are still semi-synthetic, which means that it is either based on a plant molecule or that plant substances are added to the final product at some stage of the manufacturing process.

Phytotherapy is the art of healing (oneself) with plants and vegetables. There is a correlation between the art of eating and drinking and the art of healing with the help of medicinal plants.

The plants are used in a great variety of ways:

• As products obtained after a simple manual or mechanical treatment: cut and dried plants for herb teas, decoctions, bath additives, and compresses; pulverized plants for use in capsules, etc.
• As products obtained when the active principles have been extracted by various means:
    • *The alcohols*: tinctures, mother tinctures, alcoholates.
    • *The glycerine maceration products*: mainly obtained from fresh buds, young shoots, willow catkins, etc.
    • *The syrups*, the fluid extracts, the muse, etc., which are less common.

- Finally, the products obtained through distillation:
    - The essential oils, hydrolates or floral waters, and alcoholates.

The latter bring us back again to aromatherapy, a branch of phytotherapy which has become an independent discipline in its own right due to its development and high degree of effectiveness. However, since about 1940, phytoaromatherapy has developed as a combination of both of these therapies and even gained advocates within the medical profession.

The therapy which employs phytotherapy and aromatherapy uses the many properties and possibilities of plants, permitting a far-reaching effect on all levels. Their vitalizing power acts on the organs, tissue, cells, molecules, atoms and their particles in a supportive and derivative manner. They influence the functions of the hormonal and autonomous nervous systems, as well as those of the central nervous system. They are also involved in catalysis, with an effect similar to that of the trace elements.

Chapter X

Bibliography

Phytoaromatherapy is a vast and fascinating subject at the intersection of the mineral, vegetable, animal, and human worlds with all their dimensions. This field is particularly fascinating because it is so rich and has a history which merges with our own history. Human beings have always used plants in funeral rites, religious ceremonies, for food, healing, in order to build dwellings and make tools and clothes, as well as clothing and personal hygiene.

On the other hand, since the turn of the century phytoaromatherapy has experienced an upswing as a result of research scientific investigation. The resulting findings represent a great enrichment for phytoaromatherapy.

The scope of this book does not permit us to delve more deeply into this vast field of research, which why even this brief bibliography may be useful for those who wish to learn more about this subject.

We are currently working on a larger book and research which attempts to create a synthesis of various approaches: the Eastern tradition with its Yin/Yang duality; the anthroposophical approach which connects the mineral and vegetable kingdoms with human beings and the cosmos in a unique manner; and finally, research on phytoaromatherapy in the treatment of the terrain or humoral environment, carried out mainly by the French Society for Phytotherapy and Aromatherapy.

Will a synthesis of all this be possible? Perhaps it will at least be possible to discover major factors uniting these different sources of knowledge so that we can better understand our health. This will help us restore and maintain it.

Aromatherapy
Azaloux, A.: *Contribution à l'étude de la therapeutique antiseptique par les essences végétales.* Medical thesis. Toulouse, 1943.
Bardeau, F.: *La médecine aromatique.* Ed. Laffont: Paris, 1976.
Belaiche, P.: *Traité de phytothérapie et d'aromatherapie.* 3 volumes. Ed. Maloine: Paris, 1979.
Carillon, A.: Pour un bon usage des plantes (phytothérapie, aromathérapie). Ed. Vie et Santé: Dammaire-les-Lys, (No year.)

Cazal, R.: *Contribution à l'étude de l'activité pharmacodynamique de quelques essences de labiés.* Thesis. Toulouse, 1944.
– Report of the International Congresses of the F.S.P.A. (French Society of Ph y toth erap y a nd Aromatherap y). 19, Bld. Beausejour, 75016, PARIS, FRANCE

Courmount, P., A. Morel and I. Bay, *Sur le pouvoir infertilisant de quelques essences végétables vis-à-vis du bacille tuberculeux humain.* C.R. Soc. Biology, 1927.

Couvreur, A.: Les produits aromatiques utilisées en pharmacie. Ed. Vigot: Paris, 1939.

Franchomme, P. and D. Pénoel: *L'aromathèrapie exactement.* Ed. P. Jallois: Limoges, 1990.
– *Phyto-médecine.* Published by the College of Introduction to Medicinal Plants, Paris, (no year).

Gattefossé, R.M.: *Antiseptiques essentiels* Ed. Desforges, Girardot & Cie., 1931.
– *Aromatherapie les huiles essentielles hormones végétales.* Ed. Desforges & Cie., 1931.

Gümbel, D.: *Ganzheitsmedizinishce Hauttherapie mit Heilkräuter-Essenzen.* Karl F. Haug Verlag, GmbH & Co.: Heidelberg, 2nd Edition 1984.

Henglein, M.: *Die Heilende Kraft der Wohlgerüche und utld Essenzen.* Schönberger Verlag: München, 1985.

Krack, N.: *Nasale Reflextherapie mit ätherischen Ölen.* Haug Verlag: Heidelberg, 3rd Edition 1982.

Kubeczka, H.-H.: *Ätherische Öle – Analytik, Physiologie, Zusammensetzung.* G. Thieme Verlag: Stuttgart, 1982.
– *Vorkommen und Analytik ätherischer Öle.* G. Thieme Verlag: Stuttgart, 1979.

Lagrange, J.: *Mémento d'aromathérapie vétérinaire.* Ed. Agriculture et Vie, 1979.

Leclerc, H.: *Les épices plantes condimentaires.* Ed. Masson, 1929.

Maury, M.: *Die Geheimnisse der Aromatherapie.* Windpferd Verlag: Aitrang, 2nd Edition 1991.

Moiroux, J.: Les huiles essentielles en dermatologie vétérinaire. Thesis, Lyon, 1943.

Müller, A.: *Die physiologischen und pharmakologischen Wirkungen der ätherischen Öle.* Haug Verlag: Heidelberg, 1951.

Passet, J.: *Thym vulgaris.* Thesis, Montpellier, 1971.

Porcher-Pimpard: *Contribution à l'etude du pouvoir antiseptique des essences végétales.* PhD Thesis in Pharmacy: Toulouse, 1942.

Rouvière, A. and M.-C. Meyer: *La santé par les huiles essentielles.* M.A. Edition: Paris, 1983.

Sarbach, R.: *Contribution à la désinfection des atmospheres; Etudes des proprietes antiseptiques de cinquante-quatre huiles essentielles.* PhD Thesis in Pharmacy: Rennes, 1962.

Tisserand, R.: *Aromatherapie.* Bauer Verlag: Freiburg, 4th Edition 1988.
– *Das Aromatherapie-Heilbuch.* Windpferd Verlag: Aitrang, 3rd Edition, 1992.

Valnet, J.: *Aromathérapie.* Ed. Maloine: Paris, 10th Edition, 1984.

Valnet, J., Ch. Duraffourd, J. Cl. Lapraz: *Une médecine nouvelle, Phytothérapie et Aromatherapie: comment guérir les maladies infectieuses par les plantes.* Ed. Presses de la Renaissance: Paris, 1978.

Viaud, H., J. Lamblin, J. M. Dufour: *Huiles essentielles, hydrolats.* Ed. Présence: St. Vincent-sur-Jabron, 1983.

Phytotherapy

Aurenche: *Plantes de guérison.* Ed. Legrand, 1956.

Bardeau, F.: *La pharmacie du Bon Dieu.* Ed. Laffont: Paris. (No year.)

Béranger-Beauquesne, L., M. Pinkas, and M. Torck: *Les plantes dans la therapeutique moderne.* Ed. Maloine: Paris, 1975.

Bernadet, M.: *La phyto-aromathérapie pratique.* Ed. Dangles: St. Jean-de-Braye, 1983.

Chrubasik, J.and S.: *Kompendium der Heilpflanzen.* Hippokrates Verlag: Stuttgart, 1983.

Debuigne: Le Larousse des Plantes qui guérissent. Larousse: Paris, 1975 and 1976.

Fischer, G. and E. Krug: *Heilkräuter und Arzneipflanzen.* Haug Verlag: Heidelberg, 7th Edition 1987.

Fournier, P.: *Le livre des Plantes médicinales et vénéneuses de France.* 3 volumes; Ed. P. Lechevalier, 1948.

Gäbler, H.: *Gesund durch Heilpflanzen.* Hippokrates Verlag: Stuttgart, 1979.

Lieutagui, P.: *Le livre des bonnes herbes.* Ed. Morel, 1966.

Mességué, M.: *Die Kräuter meines Vaters.* Molden Verg: Vienna, 1973.
– *Die Natur hat immer recht.* Molden Verlag: Vienna, 1973.
– *Von Menschen und Pflanzen.* Molden Verlag: Vienna, 1972.

Palaiseul, J: *Nos grands-mères savaient.* Ed Laffont: Paris. (No year.)

200

– *Tous les espoirs de guérir.* Ed. Laffont: Paris. (No year.)

Paris, R. and H. Moysé: *Précis de matière médicale.* 3 Volumes. Ed. Masson: Paris, 1965 ff.

Pelikan, W.,: *Heilpflanzezenkunde: Der Mensch and die Heilpflanzen.* 3 Volumes. Philosophisch-anthroposophischer Verlag: Dornach, 1975 ff.

Pelt, J.M.: *La médecine par les plantes.* Ed. Fayard: Paris, 1981.

Perrot, E. and R. Paris: *Les plantes médicinales.* P.U.F: Paris, 1971.

Schauenberg, P. and F. Paris: *Guide des plantes médicinales.* Ed. Delachaux & Niestlé, 1969.

Spaich, W.: *Moderne Pythotherapie.* Haug Verlag: Heidelberg, 1979.

Tetau, M. Bergeret: *La phytothérapie rénovée.* Ed. Maloine: Paris, 1972.

Treben, M: *Gesundheit aus der Apotheke Gottes.* Ennsthaler Verlag: Steyr, 1980.

Valnet, J.: *Phytothérapie.* Ed. Maloine: Paris, 1976.

Biological Medicine and Nutrition

Aubert, C.: *L'assiette aux céréales.* Ed. Terre Vivante: Paris. (No year.)

Bott, V.: *Anthroposophische Medizin.* Haug Verlag: Heidelberg, 2nd Edition 1980.

Bressy, P.: *La bielectronique et les mystères de la vie.* Ed. Le Courier du Livre: Paris. (No year.)

Buchinger, O.: *Das Heilfasten und seine Hilfsmethoden als biologischer Weg.* Hippokrates Verlag: Stuttgart, 21st Edition 1987.

Dogma, M.: Prenez en main votre santé. Ed. La Maisnie: Paris, 1979.

Dextrait, R.: *Traité de médecine naturelle. La méthode harmoniste et nombreuses autres publications.* Ed. Vivre en Harmonie: Paris. (No year.)

Elmau, H.: *Bioelektronik und Säuren-Basen-Haushalt in Theorie und Praxis.* Haug Verlag: Heidelberg, 1985.

Hasler, U.: *Eubiotik.* Haug Verlag: Heidelberg, 3rd Edition 1979.

Kollath, W.: *Die Ordnung unserer Nahrung.* Haug Verlag: Heidelberg, 13th Edition 1986.

Koob, O.: *Gesundheit – Krankheit – Heilung.* TB Fischer Verlag: Frankfurt, 3rd Edition 1987.

Kousmine, C.: *Soyez bien dans votre assiette.* Ed. Tchou: Paris, 1980.

Lützner, H.: *Wie neugeboren durch Fasten.* Verlag Gräfe und Unzer: Munich, 1980.

Marchesseau, P.V.: *Soins d'urgence par les plantes (1945) et de nombreux autres écrits.* Published and edited by the Etudes de Naturopathie: Paris, 1945.

Passebecq, A. and J.: *Votre santé par la diététique et l'alimentation saine, et d'autres publications.* Ed. Dangles, St. Jean-de-Braye. (No year.)

Renzenbrink, U.: *Ernährungskunde aus anthroposophischer Erkenntnis.* Philosophisch-anthroposophischer Verlag: Dornach, 2nd Edition 1986.

Souzenelle, A.: *Le symbolisme du corps humain.* Ed. Dangles, St. Jean-de-Braye. (No year.)

Valnet J.: Docteur Natur. Ed. Fayard: Paris, 1971.
  – Traitement des maladies par Ies légumes, les fruits et les céréales. Ed. Maloine: Paris, 1974.

About the Author

Rodolphe BALZ was born in 1944 in Geneva. After his secondary studies and university education, he was awarded his degree in Sociology and Geography—the science of the earth. He became a teacher and, with a holistic approach, has attempted to understand human beings and our relationship to our environment. He has long been interested in medicinal plants and was introduced to their uses by Swiss and French naturopaths.

For about fifteen years, Rodolphe Balz has been involved in the organic cultivation of aromatic and medicinal plants in the Drome Departement at the foot of the French Alps. This work has led to the art of obtaining essential oils through plant distillation. At the same time, he has also privately studied and investigated the therapeutic value of plants and essential oils for the treatment of human disorders. This research has extended to include veterinary medicine and plant diseases as well.

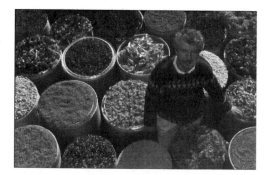

" Do not seek the Law in your Scriptures,
for the Law is alive whereas the written word is dead.
The Law is manifest in all that is alive.
You will find it
    in the grass,
    in the tree,
    in the river,
    in the mountain,
    in the birds of the sky,
    the fish of the lakes an_ ...e seas.
Yet seek it above all within yourself.
For truly I say to you:
All that is alive is closer to God
than Scriptures without life."

Essenian Gospel, Book I

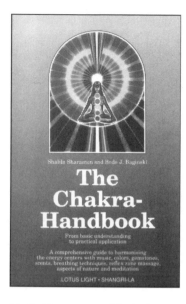

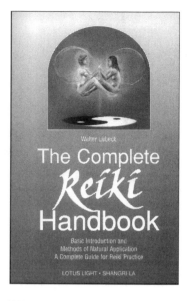

Shalila Sharamon and Bodo J. Baginski

The Chakra Handbook

From Basic Understanding to Practical Application

Knowledge of the energy centers provides us with deep, comprehensive insight into the effects the subtle powers have on the human organism. This book vividly describes the functioning of the energy centers. For practical work with the chakras this book offers a wealth of possibilities: the use of sounds, colors, gemstones, and fragrances with their own specific effects, augmented by meditation, breathing techniques, foot reflexology massage of the chakra points, and the instilling of universal life energy. The description of nature experiences, yoga practices, and the relationship of each indiviual chakra to the zodiac additionally provides inspiring and valuable insight.

192 pages, $ 14.95
ISBN 0-941524-85-X

Walter Lübeck

The Complete Reiki Handbook

Basic Introduction and Methods of Natural Application – A Complete Guide for Reiki Practice

This handbook is a complete guide for Reiki practice and a wonderful tool for the necessary adjustment to the changes inherent in a new age. The author's style of natural simplicity, much appreciated by the readers of his many bestselling books, wonderfully complements this basic method for accessing universal life energy. He shares with us, as only a Reiki master can, the personal experience accumulated in his years of practice. Lovely illustrations of the different positions make the information as easily accessible visually as the author's direct and undogmatic style of writing. This work also offers a synthesis of Reiki and many other popular forms of healing.

192 pages, $ 14.95
ISBN 0-941524-87-6

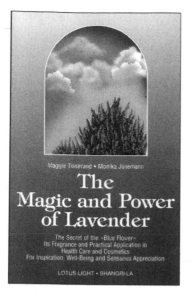

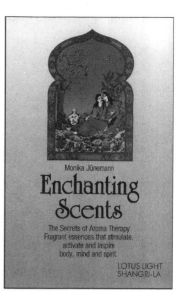

Magie Tisserand · Monika
Jünemann

The Magic and Power of
Lavender

The Secret of the Blue Flower

The scent of lavender practically has
permeated whole regions of Europe,
contributing to their special character, and dominated perfumery for
most of its history. To this very day,
lavender has remained one of the
most familiar, popular, and utilized of
all fragrances.

This book introduces you to the de-
lightful and enticing secrets of this
plant and its essence, demonstrating
its healing power, while also present-
ing the places and people involved in
its cultivation. The authors have
asked doctors, holistic health practitioners, chemists, and perfumers
about their experiences and share
them – together with their own with
you.

136 pages, $ 9.95
ISBN 0-941524-88-4

Monika Jünemann

Enchanting Scents

**The Secrets of Aromatherapy
Fragrant Essences that Stimulate,
Activate and Inspire Body, Mind
and Spirit**

Today we are just as captivated by
the magic of lovely scents and as
irresistably moved by them as ever.
The effects that essential oils have
can vary greatly. This book particularly treats their subtle influences, but
also presents and describes the
plants from which they are obtained.
It beckons you to enter the realm of
sensual experience and journey into
the world of fragrance through essences. It is an invitation to use personal scents to activate body and
spirit. Here is a key that will open your
senses to the limitless possibilities of
benefitting from fragrances as stimulants, sources of energy, and means
of healing.

128 pages, $ 9.95
ISBN 0-941524-36-1

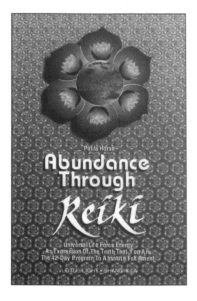

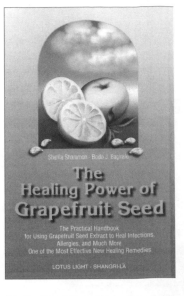

Paula Horan

Abundance Through Reiki

Universal Life Force Energy
As Expression of the Truth That
You Are
The 42-Day Program to Absolute
Fulfillment

Abundance Through Reiki is a powerful, poetic evocation of true self and universal life force energy. Its emphasis is a program of 42 steps from Core Self to Core Abundance, creating inner and outer richness. A detailed presentation in the form of two 21-day abundance plans takes you on an exploration of belief patterns that keep you from experiencing everything you need or desire.
Further topics are Reiki and abundance, abundance of health, love, friendship, knowledge, and experience. The book promotes your own natural ability to experience freedom, creativity, and authenticity.

160 pages, $14.94
ISBN 0-914955-25-X

Shalila Sharamon · Bodo J. Baginski

The Healing Power of Grapefruit Seed

The Practical Handbook for Using Grapefruit Seed Extract to Heal Infections, Allergies, and Much More. One of the Most Effective New Healing Remedies

Latest scientific studies show that plant extract from grapefruit seeds has a large range of effects and applications for both internal and external use in preventative health care, therapy, cosmetics, and baby care. Based on international research, two bestselling authors have compiled sensational therapy successes and areas of application for this biological broad spectrum therapeutic agent, antibiotic, antimycotic and antiparasitic, preservative, and hygienic agent of the future. In addition to scientific proof this practice-oriented book includes proper dosages and procedures.

160 pages, $ 12.95
ISBN 0-914955-27-6

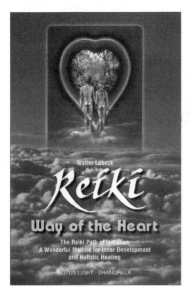

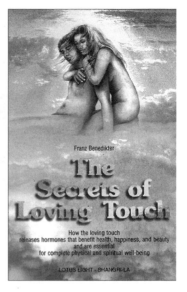

Walter Lübeck

Reiki – Way of the Heart

**The Reiki Path of Initiation
A Wonderful Method for Inner
Development and Holistic Healing**

Reiki – Way of the Heart is for everyone interested in the opportunities and experiences offered by this very popular esoteric path of perception, based on easily learned exercises conveyed by a Reiki Master to students in three degrees.

If you practice Reiki, the use of universal life energy to heal oneself and others, you will have the possibility of receiving direct knowledge about your personal development, health, and transformation.

Walter Lübeck also presents a good survey of various Reiki schools and shows how Reiki can be applied successfully in many areas of life.

208 pages, $ 14.95
ISBN 0-941524-91-4

Franz Benedikter

The Secrets of Loving Touch

**How the Loving Touch Releases
Hormones that Benefit Health,
Happiness, and Beauty and Are
Essential for Complete Physical
and Spiritual Well-Being**

Psychologist Franz Benedikter helps readers create the best possible hormonal basis for a healthy, happy, and liberated life. A release of relaxing, activating, and euphoretic hormones occurs when certain trigger zones of the body are gently touched. With this compact exercise program, we can have a positive effect on the body, mind, and soul through a form of self-massage and partner massage that is more like a loving touch. Since every healthy person has a longing to be touched, this book introduces a new age of tenderness.

144 pages, 12.95 $
ISBN 0-941524-90-6

Sources of Supply:

The following companies have an extensive selection of useful products and a long track-record of fulfillment. They have natural body care, aromatherapy, flower essences, crystals and tumbled stones, homeopathy, herbal products, vitamins and supplements, videos, books, audio tapes, candles, incense and bulk herbs, teas, massage tools and products and numerous alternative health items across a wide range of categories.

WHOLESALE:

Wholesale suppliers sell to stores and practitioners, not to individual consumers buying for their own personal use. Individual consumers should contact the RETAIL supplier listed below. Wholesale accounts should contact with business name, resale number or practitioner license in order to obtain a wholesale catalog and set up an account.

Lotus Light Enterprises, Inc.

P O Box 1008 EO
Silver Lake, WI 53170 USA
414 889 8501 (phone)
414 889 8591 (fax)
800 548 3824 (toll free order line)

RETAIL:

Retail suppliers provide products by mail order direct to consumers for their personal use. Stores or practitioners should contact the wholesale supplier listed above.

Internatural

33719 116th Street EO
Twin Lakes, WI 53181 USA
800 643 4221 (toll free order line)
414 889 8581 office phone
WEB SITE: www.internatural.com

Web site includes an extensive annotated catalog of more than 7000 products that can be ordered "on line" for your convenience 24 hours a day, 7 days a week.